HEALTH INHERITED

Dr. Adrian Bachman, DC, MS

To my wonderful wife Shawna and children Micah, Audrey, Kaden, Brynlee, and Treyson.

CONTENTS

INTRODUCTION

What are you passing on to your children?

I CONSTANTLY HEAR people asking, "Why are my children so sick? Why does it seem like they get over one thing, and then they're getting sick all over again?"

When I was a kid in grade school, I never remember them closing school because too many children were sick and they were afraid it would spread. Today, we can look at our children and see their decreased brain function. The children today are becoming overweight at such a young age with no real turnaround. Does this make you stop and think that there may be a problem?

It can also be said that more children are suffering neurological deficiencies than ever before. The term 'autism spectrum' wasn't really on anyone's mind twenty years ago. Now, it's at the forefront of struggles for many families, leaving a question in our minds of where it came from and why it is gaining incidence so quickly. The dependency on neurological medications is higher than ever, and the performance of these medications continues to decrease in most individuals over time. These are not new facts, and shouldn't be something that you are hearing for the first time.

In this book, we will look into the changes that have happened over time, getting a reality check on what we are providing our families—things we may not even know about.

"WHY DO WE CALL IT 'ALTERNATIVE MEDICINE' WHEN IT'S THE "ORIGINAL MEDICINE" THAT HUMANS HAVE USED FOR THOUSANDS OF YEARS? 'MODERN MEDICINE' WAS ONLY DISCOVERED 100 YEARS AGO!"

UNKNOWN

Many that read this may simply say that I do not truly understand what a house with a child who is "sick" with the above situation is even like. But I have to say that I do understand, because I was there at one point. This struggle is real, and I can relate. As I progressed to a better, healthier life, I was determined to help other children be able to have the same. Once I started talking to more and more families, sincerely asking why they were having these struggles with their child—whether it was being sick all the time, a lack of energy, depression/anxiety, decreased performance in school, or more increased symptoms of neurological deficits such as ADD, ADHD, autism, or behavioral issues—the story was always very similar. What they were eating had a lasting impact on how they were feeling and what they were doing.

I know some of you have already written this off, saying "my child was born this way" and denying that what they eat affects their child's situation. You are exactly right; your child's situation is not directly caused by food. However, it is important to remember that all development begins some-where. Our children are exposed to what we take in during the crucial developmental phase while they are in the womb or even preconception. Now, don't start blaming yourself for this either, as you might have followed the recommended standard diets and did what you could to eat healthy. But did you really know every aspect of what was in the prepared meal you were eating? Most didn't, so don't start degrading yourself for your children's results. Instead, use this time to make a difference and enhance their minds for a brighter future.

I have to state that not all symptoms that our children experience or even what we go through as adults is directly caused by what we eat. However, it does play a large role, and it's what you do to make the change in your children's lives that will turn them around and help them explore the very best life they can have going forward. Making this change can be the beginning of a new generation that is passed on for many generations to come.

As you continue reading this book, I want you to try to absorb as much information as you possibly can and reflect upon it for yourself, your family, and your children. I also encourage you to become an advocate for your children and their friends and family as well. Remember, the change in one single life can make a huge impact on the entire world. Why not let this basic information be the start to make that change? I urge you to reflect on the simple steps that can change your life.

Eating right and becoming as nutritious as you can for your family is simple, especially as you implement this into your daily life and it moves from a "diet" to a lifestyle change. It then becomes fun and you will quickly start to see the improvements. I hope you will enjoy sharing this lifestyle with everyone you come in contact with. I personally challenge you to pass it on, start a new trend, and build a community around this new lifestyle you are creating for your family.

No, not everything you read will resonate with you, and not every tip will apply to your situation. But even if you gain just a little nugget of information, I hope this book will give you that next step you are looking for to empower yourself, your family, and the world. Just stop and think—what would happen if we could enhance the minds of all the children in our school, community, state, or the world? What great things could come of this? It's as simple as changing what and how you eat and joining your kids in the process.

EATING RIGHT AND BECOMING AS NUTRITIOUS AS YOU CAN FOR YOUR FAMILY IS SIMPLE, ESPECIALLY AS YOU IMPLEMENT THIS INTO YOUR DAILY LIFE AND IT MOVES FROM A "DIET" TO A LIFESTYLE CHANGE. IT THEN BECOMES FUN AND YOU WILL QUICKLY START TO SEE THE IMPROVEMENTS.

Without any further ado, let's get to the point and discover what needs to be done. I assure you that I will try my best to be as transparent as I can, giving you all of the details and leaving nothing out. I want the world to know how easy this is and what little effort it takes to be the very best "you" that you can be. The first chapter is going to spell out the discouraging statistics, and then I will break it down by topic and explain what can be done to improve these declining health numbers. Then, it will be on you to make that first step and implement the change that will help your children and family. If for any reason you have additional questions or don't completely understand something, please feel free to reach out to me. I'll be more than happy to help you along the way to see you and your family succeed. Remember, we are in this together for the lifestyle we all deserve. Are you ready?

"The greatest medicine of all
is to teach people not to need it."

- Hippocrates

1

EPIDEMIC

"Why are our children so sick?"

WHY ARE WE LESS healthy today than ever, yet we are so much more advanced in our knowledge of health? Nearly every American is taking some sort of pharmaceutical drug or supplement, yet the life expectancy of our children is shorter than it is for the parents. What is wrong with this picture? Simply stated, we have forgotten to use the simple things that God has given us to be truly healthy. We forget to "let food be thy medicine and medicine by thy food." If we are lacking in a vitamin, let us eat the foods that give us those vitamins. If we lack vitamin D, go outside. If we have aches and pains, use plant-based essential oils. It really can be that simple!

Epidemic! Pandemic! Endemic! Call it whatever you want when it comes to the health and wellness of our children and families. It doesn't matter where you look, there is a rise in childhood diseases in many countries—but especially the United States. Even if we don't look at the numbers and simply look around, we can see that the stature and appearance of many around us is much larger than we once were. The same can be said with the sicknesses around us that are driven by our poor diets and sedentary lifestyles.

This has dramatically changed over the years, and more than ever we have found our children and families not moving, but rather being willing to sit around and do nothing to improve their overall health. Obesity and diabetes alone have increased at an astounding rate and are affecting kids today at younger and younger ages. This all stems from the lack of activity and the convenience of processed and prepared foods. Even the portions kids eat today are much larger than they once were, and that hasn't aided this systemic disease process that has affected them.

Many may grow bored and prefer not to be consumed with all the numbers that go along with this, but I think in order to see why our health is inherited and why it is so important to establish good habits in our children, we have to be honest with ourselves and face the reality of numbers that tell the story. Now, we can argue that numbers don't show the entire picture, and this can be true. However, consider the numbers that are statistically presented to you here and then stop for a moment and look around you when you are out and about. Even further, look at your own household and see what your family is honestly doing and how they are going about it. Really be honest with yourself and evaluate what is going on. Are your children playing and eating the same way you did as a child? Are they as active, or do they enjoy the conveniences of modern technology that have replaced the time we spent doing physical activities? This isn't here to deter you from the benefits of having something easier in our lives. This is simply to recognize that even though technology and conveniences have replaced physical activity, it doesn't mean we can sit around and not improve our health.

This means that now, more than ever, we need to be moving and consciously doing something physical to increase our heart rate for a period of time, improving the oxygen exchange in our body.

"THE FOOD YOU EAT CAN EITHER BE THE SAFEST AND MOST POWERFUL FORM OF MEDICINE . . . . OR THE SLOWEST FORM OF POISON."
ANN WIGMORE

Recently we have found ourselves in a point where we have been more isolated from everyone than ever, and while that has its own extreme negatives in our mental cognition with the lack of connection with others, it has also led to a dramatic decrease in the physical activity of others. At first, when people were bored, there was an increase in families getting out and walking and biking more; after a period of time of isolation, they couldn't take it much longer. But once life returns a little more to normal, everyone falls back into that realm of inactivity and it makes you wonder what kids are doing today if they are not active. Growing up, it used to be that on summer evenings you could hear kids' voices all over town, and they would be out playing. Have you ever noticed that now, if you are outside on a summer evening, it can be very quiet? So, what happened to all the children and families?

It happens in our house all the time—when the children aren't active, they become bored. When they become bored, they look for things to eat to fill their time. When they get something to eat, they get sleepy, and the cycle continues on and on, answering the question of why we have the obesity and disease rate we do today. We as a family have to get out and force ourselves to be physically active for periods of time throughout the day. This is for the wellbeing and health of our children and is not a negative thing. You can improve the outcome of your children's wellness by teaching them the importance of the body working properly. As you will discover in the exercise section of this book, we don't have to always be physically active outside, as many of the activities can be done right in our home. However, when able, it is crucial to get them outside along with ourselves, allowing them to get fresh air and sun as much as possible. Having the ability for both them and ourselves to deeply inhale the oxygen-rich air that fills our lungs enhances the ability to make that oxygen and carbon dioxide exchange in our lungs and our blood. Just picture it: the older we get, the more tired and less enthusiastic we are to get up and get moving. Our blood becomes old in our bodies the same way and needs to have that proper exchange to be able to get the new oxygen in and the old out, allowing us to function as we should. We are definitely thankful for our homes, but they come with their own set of toxins and restrictions, keeping us confined and not allowing us to make that fresh oxygen exchange in our bodies. This is not just in the Midwest of the United States, but everywhere. Thus, it is so important to get outside and get that fresh air!

ACCORDING TO THE CENTER FOR DISEASE CONTROL (CDC), IT HAS BEEN RECORDED THAT THERE ARE 13.7 MILLION CHILDREN AND ADOLESCENTS SUFFERING FROM OBESITY.

According to the Center for Disease Control (CDC) it has been recorded that there are 13.7 million children and adolescents suffering from obesity. This can be affected by ethnicity, demographics, and socioeconomic status across the United

States. However, there is one thing that is the same: if we can get our children to eat right and remove the large amounts of processed foods and toxins entering into their bodies, it would drive up their ability to fight off this obesity. Then we can increase their activity, which will also drive down the obesity rate.

If you follow the trends from the past couple of years to the past decade, you will see these rates continue to go up steadily with no decline. So, if we add another year to this, what will the overall outcome be for these children? Then take the same 13.7 million kids that are obese today, and imagine that they don't change their habits—and it would be extremely rare if they did because they do what they see and what is provided to them—what will they be like 10, 15, or 20 years from now? That is why our diseases are also on the rise and affecting our children at a much younger rate.

Obesity can lead to type two diabetes and poor sugar regulation. It also increases the risk of cancer and behavioral issues caused by a lack of proper nutrition and wellness in our children. It is a cycle that we can easily fall into. If we don't alter the outcome of our younger generations and stop the traditional effect of how they eat and exercise, these numbers will continue to go up. If we can alter the family mindset and make a lifestyle change, we have the potential to help them learn, bringing down the statistics and changing the outcome for children and adults alike.

We've discussed that in the United States we have an increase in obesity, but let's look at the world as a whole. We must face the facts that this issue isn't just one region or another, but is worldwide, and this information affects everyone in the world. It was said that from 1990 until 2016, there was a jump in early childhood obesity from 32 million to 41 million worldwide for those up to age five. What about the remaining ages up to eighteen? This is a number that none of us could actually comprehend. We also overlook the fact that not all children get counted, so think of the reality of the number of children that are affected by this. This can affect the epigenetics of children and adults, but we have to know that much of this obesity can be controlled. Obesity is only one problem in our children, but is one of the largest problems that affects so many children today, and it leads to most of the diseases that our children are faced with. If one isn't affected by disease as a child or teen, they certainly will have a high risk of being affected at a later age with high blood pressure, cardiovascular disease, stroke, cancer, and the list can go on and on.

Once again, you don't have to believe the numbers that are presented, but you can look around you, no matter what country you are in, and see for yourself. Kids are much larger and less able to move around than they once were. We have to figure out a way to improve these number, and unfortunately, there is no easy pill that can fix this. We have to educate ourselves and start at home, teaching our children the importance of eating right and living an active lifestyle. These numbers aren't going to change unless we all take an active role.

Let's start now by reviewing what you read, making simple changes little by little, and you will start to see a difference. Then, start to share with others and help them to see that the best outcomes come from changing our mind and making a lifestyle change.

There is another focus and a few more numbers that need to be considered when talking about children and how their diet plays a large role in their overall performance and outcome: The research and behavioral information that Dr. Robert Melillo has spent many years focusing on, and the connection between the brain and what has driven up the neurological childhood diseases. Based on his work, it was referenced that approximately 21 million children are affected by a neurological deficiency of some kind, which can include behavioral issues, ADD, ADHD, autism, dyslexia, and many others that affect the brain function of our children. One can have many different thought processes about where those come from, which can include the immunization of these kids or the foods the mother consumed while pregnant. As all of these theses could be potentially true and are well supported, it can also stem from the foods our kids are putting in their mouths and the lack of activity to stimulate their brains, causing degeneration.

> **THE QUESTION THAT WE NEED TO SPEND SOME TIME THINKING ABOUT IS, WHERE DO THESE FOODS COME FROM? HOW PURE WERE THEY WHEN THEY WERE HARVESTED, AND HOW GOOD CAN THEY BE FOR OUR BODY? WHEN PLACED IN A CAN, DO THEY PICK UP THE HEAVY METALS THAT ARE FOUND IN THE CAN, OR ARE THEY CLEAN AND EASILY DIGESTIBLE FOR OUR BODY?**

We have so many foods that are convenient to use today, foods that are pre-packaged and ready to eat. We even have foods that are good for us where we can open a can and dump them out, consuming them in minutes. The question that we need to spend some time thinking about is: Where do these foods come from? How pure were they when they were harvested, and how good can they be for our body? When placed in a can, do they pick up the heavy metals that are found in the can, or are they clean and easily digestible for our body? When a mother is pregnant, did she prepare her body by cleansing all the toxins and heavy metals, preparing the right environment for the developing child? When these children are born, are they getting the right exposure to the good bacteria during birth from the mother? Some of these things we cannot control, and it should never be placed on the mother to assume responsibility for things that are out of her control. We have to face the facts and truly be honest with ourselves about whether these environments have been the best for our kids early on or not.

Once we understand this, then we can look at what our children are growing up with, how our family dynamics may play a role in it all, and what we can change. Frequently, before one can realize that their child has been affected by a neurological condition, they are of school age and about 6-7 years have already passed. Was the diet filled with convenience, leaving them slurping on dyed fruit punch and soda or eating pre-packaged foods? Were they consuming plenty of water to flush out all the toxins that might be building up? Were they living in an old house that might have increased lead paint, allowing them to suck or lick things that might have given them a possibility to be exposed? These are all things that we must consider, not to make us feel we are bad parents, but to bring to our attention and realize that we maybe didn't know that this could alter our children's outcome. We aren't going out to the garden anymore, plucking fresh vegetables to eat, and in many cases our children aren't playing outside and getting exposed to many of the good bacteria and the lifestyle that they need to flourish and grow. We can see how these toxin-filled exposures can creep in, and we have to address them and see what we can do to flush them out, helping their brains to fully function as they are. We may have to get them heading in the right direction and guide them so that we can enhance their insides, allowing them to get those good neurological connections firing and improve their outcome.

This has been tested and tried over and over again as we try to find ways to enhance the brain function of our children, and the best way is to provide good foods to heal the gut and enhance the brain via those connections leading to the gut and the brain. Then, focus on improving the brain stimulation and enhance learning through creativity and productivity. These can all be brought together and help turn our struggling children with these types of neurological deficits around, giving them normal lives they can enjoy.

It must be stated that this in no way is designed to treat a child or even diagnose them, but simply a guide to help you encourage your family to eat well and function to the best ability possible. At this point, some of you may feel discouraged about what we have done to make our children the way they are and wonder how can we fix our mistakes. This is in no way a book designed to make you feel guilty about how to raise your children or to say that what you did maybe led them to a neurological condition. Remember, many of these things are out of our control. We have to remember that God is in ultimate control, and we can only do what we know and have been taught. Hopefully, having a guide moving forward will help us be better at raising a healthy family, but it in no way can control the outcome of God's plan for our family. Always remember He is always in ultimate control, and we can only do what we can to the best of our ability. So many times, families try to create miracles in their dietary and family lifestyles, causing increased stress on the mother or family as a whole, soon causing everyone to be in despair and preventing a full outcome to be completed. Remember, as a parent you can only do what you can do, and can only support with the resources that you have available to you as a family. Leave it at that, and do the very best you can, making the best of what you have available to you.

Let's face it, we all want the very best for our family, and we will do everything we can to make sure we give the very best to our family. At the end of the day, the simple knowledge of eating right, getting good exercise, drinking plenty of water, and sleeping right is the daily function that we can pass on to our children for years to come. So many plans contain complex methods we have to follow, and we simply cannot imagine implementing them into our family. As a result they never get done. We are busy raising families, and some days it seems that we continue to get busier and busier, not allowing enough time to do all we want to do. Making major changes in our family's lifestyle that take even more complexity and time than we have will not lead us to success in the end. We know that we cannot add anything more than what we already are doing to our life, so we aren't as willing to implement these changes even though we know we need to.

One thing should be considered: that everything we do should be simple, and something done already in the tasks we are already doing. This means that we shouldn't re-invent the wheel if it is already working for us in a functional way. Just find ways you can implement these nutritional lifestyles without changing what you are already doing. That is how it can be simple—use what you have, stop worrying about the little things, and look at the big picture. As you travel through this book, you will see that nutritional wellness doesn't have to mean every single item gets measured out, or putting your kids on a scale every day to monitor their progress. Simply live, do your best, and make the changes you can, and you will see outcomes. It may not happen in a day or week, but throughout months to years you will make a difference, and when that happens you can look back and truly feel you did all you could for your family.

"You don't have to cook fancy or complicated
masterpieces; just good food from fresh ingredients."
- Julia Child

2

DIET

You are what you eat!

WHEN IT COMES TO changing your family and instilling core nutritional values into your children to be inherited for years to come, it all starts with the diet. Don't think of the term "diet" here as a quick weight loss program in the traditional form, but as a diet in the sense of what we eat during our entire life. The first issue with many of the diets today is that they are very successful if followed to the exact point. It doesn't matter what diet you are on, and we all know that there are a lot of them out there. Consider how many you have tried personally and roped your family into joining you in your adventure. It worked, and you were going to get yourself into shape and your family healthy. How long this did last? For most, it can last for a while, and then it fades away because you cheat here or do badly there. In the end, you count your losses and decide you'll try to do the best that you can, but know that it won't be successful all the time.

This is the story that I hear over and over, and one I have experienced myself. When one diets, in the back of your mind you feel that one day in the future you will go back to eating what you want, when you want it, and it leads you to reach this goal sooner than you plan. Everyone wants to eat what they want when they want and if we had our way we would indulge in cereal, pizza, cookies, ice cream, pop, and candy every single day. Maybe not that bad, but you understand that the "bad" food is so much easier to convince ourselves to eat than what is good and nutritionally sound for us. Instead of doing a quick weight-loss program and then going back to normal, we have to realize and show our children how dieting affects our gut's microbiome and what damaging effects it has on our bodies' function over time. The see-saw effect of eating well and going back to unhealthy food is not healing our gut and supporting our overall health and wellness at all.

"WHEN YOU START EATING FOOD WITHOUT LABELS, YOU NO LONGER NEED TO COUNT CALORIES."

AMANDA KRAFT

So, what do we do to become successful for ourselves and for our family? That is the hardest part, but it starts with changing one's mindset. We have to change our traditional thinking and know ourselves and our bad habits the most. We have to address these nutritional modifications as a lifestyle change. When we start to understand and realize what all the traditional convenience foods do to our body's gut and organs, it makes it much easier to stay away from them.

When we continually eat foods that don't support our gastrointestinal tract, we continue to break down the lining of the gut. This lining protects the gastrointestinal tract contents from being exposed to the bloodstream until they are broken down enough to pass through and be beneficial to the blood cells. When we weaken our gastrointestinal lining, we weaken the passageway between the gut and the bloodstream. When this happens, it causes larger particles to pass through and inflames the lining along with the intestinal wall because foreign objects have been introduced to the system. These foreign intruders are bacteria, larger proteins, or any other pathogen that can skip across this membrane layer. When the lining becomes inflamed, it then causes mucus to develop to protect it from these foreign invaders. This mucus acts as a guard, not allowing the small particles to pass through—which are the good nutrients that we need. This leads to malabsorption because we don't get the good vitamins and minerals from the foods we eat and the supplements we take.

If we continue to eat like this meal after meal, we'll never let this inflammation in the lining improve and heal, along with removal of that mucus that has built up. That will get excreted over time, allowing the good nutrients to pass through. This continued damage will then alter the communication that we have between the brain and the gut through the enteric system, which is the neurological system in our gastrointestinal tract. This enteric system tells the brain to release enzymes and bile to break down our foods. When we hinder this from working properly because of the inflammation in the gastrointestinal lining, we don't release these valuable tools to break down our foods. This subsequently leads to fermentation in the gut, especially with more complex proteins, which does further damage to the digestive system. That damage inhibits the transmission of neurological impulses back to the brain through the vagus nerve and the brain also doesn't get the valuable nutrients it needs to function. This reduces the overall ability of the brain to operate at a level that is needed, and is why many suffer from brain dysfunction when their gastrointestinal tract isn't working. It can also cause constipation or diarrhea, along with burping and flatulence.

Stop calling the way you eat a "diet", and referring to it as a diet that you have your whole family on. It will make your children very uncomfortable and rebel against eating what is good and healthy for you, particularly if you go out with your family and friends and make a big deal about your family not being able to eat what is being served by packing all your own food for the occasion. You can be assured that you now have a diet plan for the family and not a lifestyle change. Your children won't buy into this method, and soon, no matter how hard you try to keep them from eating unhealthy food, you will find them sneaking cookies and sweets to satisfy their cravings. Stop calling it a diet, and stop bringing attention to it. Make

THE FIRST STEP INTO MAKING A LIFESTYLE CHANGE IS TO UNDERSTAND THAT THERE HAS TO BE AN ANALYSIS MADE TO SEE WHERE YOU ARE AS A FAMILY AND WHERE YOU CAN IMPROVE. IT GOES WITHOUT SAYING THAT WE ALL HAVE A GOOD IDEA OF WHAT WE SHOULD BE EATING AND WHAT FOODS ARE BEST LEFT IN THE GARBAGE CAN, NEVER TO ENTER THE HOUSE AGAIN.

these lifestyle changes that seem normal and don't stand out, rather than making your family look like they are self-isolated and different from everyone.

This would be the first step at becoming successful in making great changes to your family's nutritional plan. Of course, there are always the exceptions. A child or possibly the whole family does have a major health problem or another reason why they need to bring their own food, and this of course is

100% acceptable and encouraged. But the difference you must understand is that we need to eat whole healthy foods on a daily basis for our overall health and wellness. But when we go out and about, we do our very best to choose the healthy options that are offered and leave the rest without making a big disturbance about it.

The first step into making a lifestyle change is to understand that there has to be an analysis made to see where you are as a family and where you can improve. It goes without saying that we all have a good idea of what we should be eating and what foods are best left in the garbage can, never to enter the house again. We have to sit down with our family and talk this over, helping them all to understand—including our spouses—and get everyone on board. They should know that those chips may not be in the cupboard in the future for a snack, but there will be a replacement that they can grab and utilize where they are hungry. If you cannot help educate or at least get everyone on the same level to truly understand what is needed to follow through with the nutritional support, it will make your job much harder, and in the end will look more like that fad diet everyone else is trying to get thin on. The main goal with working with your entire family is to help them see the benefits and truly understand that this is the right way we should be eating, because we'll feel so much better. This is how Grandma and Grandpa used to eat and their parents ate—whole foods, not the pre-packaged processed stuff that makes it so convenient to cook.

Depending on what stage your family is in, you might struggle getting older children to see where you're going with this and have them buy in to the ideas. Sometimes teenage children really have a hard time with the changes that are made in their family, mentioning over and over that they are eating weird and funny.

But with time and patience, and by explaining the difference that various foods have on your body and what negative effects they will have by eating conveniently now, over time they can grasp and truly understand that they will feel better when they eat well. Speaking from experience, they will realize that when they eat junk food, they become tired and struggle to get up in the morning, get acne, or just overall feel "yucky". They wanted it for the moment–and it sounded good–but shortly after, they didn't want any part of it and would rather grab fruit or vegetables as a snack.

This isn't something that should be forced on them. But if you continually provide a loving environment where there are fresh fruits and vegetables available at all times for snacks when they are hungry, your family will start to crave the good foods and want those. They have to experience the difference for themselves to be convinced that it is real and something they want to do. Then they will convince their peers, too.

There is one thing you do not want to do, and that is to force a food change on your children and make them eat things they don't want to eat. Sure, there will be times when a new vegetable could be introduced, and you try to get them to taste it, but forcing them to eat things they refuse to eat will drive them away and they will build a wall up around healthy eating. Likewise, if you put all junk foods on a "never to be consumed" list, this can lead them to secretly indulging in large amount of them behind your back. This will work against you in the end and your hard work at home will become ineffective as they will hide more than you think and won't conform to what you are trying to introduce.

Remember, this isn't a new concept we are bringing in, but one that used to be the normal in our grandparents' generation and before. One that has slipped away because of modern conveniences. We are only trying to bring our families back to the basics and remove what can be harmful for them helping them naturally heal what might be damaged and feel better. If we can start introducing the whole healthy foods to them at a young age, they will develop a palate for them.

"Do you have any cucumbers around here?" a three-year-old little guy asked his grandma. If they have these foods readily available that's what they will ask for and want. When children can feel the difference for themselves in the food choices, they will be set to go out and about and still be able to eat well, knowing it is their choice and not what Dad and Mom are making them do. It is a much more powerful example for their friends when they themselves make healthy food choices and don't eat the ice cream or drink the pop because they don't want it, rather than if their friends look on them with pity because their parents said they can't have it.

IT IS A MUCH MORE POWERFUL EXAMPLE FOR THEIR FRIENDS WHEN THEY THEMSELVES MAKE HEALTHY FOOD CHOICES AND DON'T EAT THE ICE CREAM OR DRINK THE POP BECAUSE THEY DON'T WANT IT, RATHER THAN IF THEIR FRIENDS LOOK ON THEM WITH PITY BECAUSE THEIR PARENTS SAID THEY CAN'T HAVE IT.

Is it starting to click how health can be inherited? Each family is different, and each family will deal with their individual challenges. Some of you will read this far and say that you can't do this, and that it isn't worth the time and effort. This is understandable, but as the old saying goes, "Rome wasn't built in a day." Our lifestyle changes shouldn't be made overnight, but done in a time frame that your family can work with.

Guilt! That will be one of the biggest struggles that you may face within yourself while trying to make the changes you want in your family when it comes to nutrition. Don't be too hard on yourself, and realize that every little step can be a big step in the end; we have to make those big steps in order to reach the bigger goals. Don't lose focus of this, and take these little steps one at a time by removing one item off your grocery list that doesn't support your family's healthy eating. Don't start with that hot item that your family craves each week. Start with one item that is smaller, or even simply remove the extra sugar in the diet at first. Replace the sugar in your diet with the natural sweeteners like honey or maple syrup and give that a try for a bit. Set out little steps each week and build on that. Don't come in like a hurricane and dismantle the food life your family depends on. So many families lose hope because they try to implement huge changes all at once, and it doesn't work that way. Work on little changes, adding more and more as you go. Some days you may make great advances, and other days you might take a step back. Always remember this is a lifestyle change, not a diet.

One way to begin to approach the task of changing the life-style that you currently live in (one of processed foods that contain high levels of sugar and high fructose corn syrup) is to realize how much your family is consuming as a whole. How do you honestly do this in the fairest way possible? Start by keeping a food journal and write down what goes on your family's table or what snacks are eaten on a daily basis. At the end of this book, there will be a sample chart that you can use for the next seven days to write down everything you and your family put into their mouths throughout the day. If it is candy, write it down; if it is a cookie, write it down. Everything goes down on this chart if you honestly want to know how you are doing. If someone in the family puts it in their mouth, write it down.

So many times, you might ask someone what they eat, and they tell you what you might want to hear. Or we forget what we really eat and put into our mouths on a regular basis. This has happened over and over, and it may surprise you when you find out how bad your family might be. We live in a society of convenience, and with that convenience we have many unnatural and processed things in our diet. That's the fact we have been dependent upon, and now it is showing its ill effects in increased illnesses and children suffering from more and more disease at a much younger age.

"THINK ABOUT IT, IF THERE IS A HEALTH FOOD SECTION IN THE GROCERY STORE, WHAT DOES THAT MAKE THE REST OF THE FOOD SOLD THERE?"
DR. MARK HYMAN

Once you have browsed through your kitchen and seen what you have in your cabinets as far as food, write down everything you are consuming on a daily basis as a family. Stop to really decide and set goals for the change you want to make. Don't make this complicated or stressful. A family can accomplish a lifestyle change when things are simple and straightforward. There are so many different diets and nutritional programs that want you to record everything for a long period of time or measure everything out, which then drives a busy lifestyle and creates a plan that isn't successful; we don't have time to do all these steps. Remember, this lifestyle is about taking it back to the basics and staying there, allowing you to grow and flourish in your family's wellness for years to come.

Start by removing any items that shouldn't be in your house, and don't continue to put them on your grocery list. Design basic meals that have the core components of fresh vegetables, fruits, lean meat, nuts, and seeds. That is it! If you consume a lot of diary, sugar, or grains/wheat, consider taking several weeks to slowly pull these out of your diet. They are foods that can drive inflammation and need to be eliminated. It is always best to set a goal of how long you will need to do this. Lifestyle changes are for life, so as much as possible in our own homes, we should only have the foods that support a healthy microbiome.

If your gut microbiome is fed the nutrients it needs on a daily basis to stay healthy, it will be able to successfully process a treat once in a while when you are out and about with others. This just should never become the norm in your daily life at home. In order to make these changes a lifestyle, we also have to have accessibility to freely go about our life and not have to haul a trailer-load of food with us wherever we go. It is how much we consume on a daily basis that makes the huge difference. Would a little dairy from time to time really hurt you? No, it won't hurt you if it can be processed with plenty of time to work through the digestive system and your gut isn't bombarded with it several times a day. It's when we consume it three or more times a day that it begins to cause problems, over time increasing the risk of inflammation and irritating the gastrointestinal lining, causing leakage of the nutrients that we really need. Once it starts to get irritated and we continue to consume more and more, it just causes the irritation to rise, leading to a dysfunctional gastrointestinal tract and a whole host of other problems at the bottom of the pyramid of diseases.

When our gastrointestinal tract starts to be dysfunctional, it leads to improper operation of all the organs that surround the intestines. Most importantly, it eventually will affect the brain which has a direct connection to the gut via the vagus nerve. One might not think they're really affected by what their gut is doing, but when you pull the irritants out of the diet and allow the gastrointestinal tract to properly heal, you can realize how much of a difference these had on your body. Some of these symptoms can be present in both adults and children, and we don't notice them until they are completely gone from our life. They can include burping, flatulence, headaches, stomach discomfort, constipation, diarrhea, fatigue, mood swings, behavior issues, depression, anxiety, lack of motivation, overconsumption of foods, hunger, increased temperature, stomach bloating, and many others depending on the person and their age. One can get a lot of allergy testing or have a gastrointestinal scope done to see what is going on. But why wouldn't you try to do everything you can on your own to help eliminate the issue first and not put yourself or your child through all the excessive testing? Remove the common irritants like sugar, processed foods, and dairy to see if the problems dissipate before you take drastic measures to fix the problem.

SO MANY WILL GET TEST AFTER TEST TO TRY TO FIGURE OUT THE PROBLEM. IN THE END, THEY END UP GETTING MEDICATION TO FIX AN ISSUE THAT COULD BE STEMMING FROM THEIR FOOD CONSUMPTION AND THE DAMAGE THEIR BODY IS SUCCUMBING TO.

So many will get test after test to try to figure out the problem. In the end, they end up getting medication to fix an issue that could be stemming from their food consumption and the damage their body is succumbing to. The key ingredients that be on your list to eliminate first should include, sugar, dairy, wheat, beef, and pork. Once again, don't try to eliminate them from your diet all at one time, but take them out slowly; and when you do, don't bring them back. Leave them out for good or for a period. Once you have these completely out of your diet, then start the clock and keep them completely out for a period of 90 days.

Can you handle something for just 90 days? I know some of you may say that's too long, but once you start this challenge, take it day by day and try to keep it going for as long as you can. If you bring it in one time, it may not affect you, but it brings down your guard and you start to slip up, saying you did it once so why does it matter. Keep it out of your family's consumption for the full 90 days. It is possible, as it has been done over and over, and neither you nor your family will die because of it. It may take you a month to officially get those core ingredients out of your diet, but there are so many alternatives that it shouldn't be an issue to keep them gone for good. But remember, this is only for the next 90 days.

"IT'S NOT THAT I CAN'T EAT THAT.
I'M MAKING THE HEALTHIER CHOICE NOT TO."
UNKNOWN

Make a calendar, have a paper chain, whatever you need for your family to reach the goal you have set up. You will be able to tell the difference over time if you are honest and consistent with this plan. Why is it 90 days? Because we cannot always see nutritional changes or benefits in just a week or two. You must have a long enough period to remove these negative substances or toxins from your digestive system and allow it to rebuild with the good nutrients it needs to really heal. At the same time, if you support your system with a good probiotic, multivitamin, and omega 3s, (which are further discussed in a later chapter) you can simultaneously introduce the good bacteria back into the gastrointestinal tract and allow the inflammation to decrease and the gut to heal fully. If you were only to do this for a month, you wouldn't completely remove toxins from your system and the inflammation would still have the potential to be present and flare up again, preventing you from experiencing the true difference of a healthy gut compared to a leaky or unhealthy gut. This also will allow that connection between the brain and the gut to heal, allowing your brain to get the full nutrients from the good foods that we're eating to help heal it as well, increasing our cognitive function.

Another point one could consider is that if you do something for 90 days, it will have long become a habit, and we don't desire to go back to those bad habits of ice cream before bed. We have established a good pattern and we can actually naturally continue this for life if we choose. That is a lifestyle change, and once you see the changes it brings about in your life and your family's life, you will want to continue this.

A question that always comes up is, "What do I do when we are out and about with other people and we don't want to stand out or look funny?" This makes sense, especially with children, who don't want to look out of place or weird in front of their friends or have anyone confront them about this weird way they are eating. It's fine if they know it is okay to take a small amount of something they wouldn't normally have, as long as you set the example for them that they go for the naturally healthier things, such as more vegetables or salad instead of the extra meat and potatoes. In these circumstances and only in these circumstances would you want to really consume a very small portion of maybe the meat or another item that might not be what you traditionally eat, but also heap their plate with what is available that is good for them. Nobody will really notice this if they do this on their own and don't draw attention to it. If you can pass on these items without much attention being drawn to you, then why not do so?

SO MANY ASK, "CAN I HAVE THIS OR THAT?" WHEN IT COMES TO SUCH QUESTIONS, TRY TO VISUALLY DIVIDE THE INGREDIENT DOWN TO THE PORTION YOU MIGHT CONSUME AND REALIZE THAT YOU ARE GETTING A VERY SMALL AMOUNT. THESE ARE THE LITTLE THINGS WE DON'T WANT TO OVERCONSUME OURSELVES WITH AND COMPLICATE THE PROCESS.

Ultimately, consuming a very small portion of what we might consider something we shouldn't eat can sometimes be much better than drawing attention to ourselves, leaving us and our children feeling deprived in the end, and feeling like trying live a healthy lifestyle isn't worth it. If we do that, our children will especially want to either rebel against the whole thing or give it up altogether when they come to an age where they feel free to do so. This will lessen their ability to do this long term and they'll be less successful in the end. If this happens occasionally during the month, then in the end it really won't be that big of a deal to the body and it can adapt without much trouble. The same goes for those things like condiments such as dressing, or if someone puts some cheese or sour cream on something. You don't have spent hours dissecting it or trying to remove it because it isn't something that you should have, but rather politely eat a small amount if you can't easily avoid it and move on. After all, if you were to break down that small amount of butter or diary in that larger amount of food, would you really be consuming that much? Consider that a tablespoon of butter on a pot of beans doesn't break down to that much per individual serving. The same thing can be for dressing or any of these extras.

So many ask, "Can I have this or that?" When it comes to such questions, try to visually divide the ingredient down to the portion you might consume and realize that you are getting a very small amount. These are the little things we don't want to overconsume ourselves with and complicate the process. We sometimes need these little extras to get down our Brussels sprouts or cauliflower, and it is better that you get them in with a little butter than to be eating veggies that are drowning in a cheese sauce or cream soup. Sure, you could always serve the veggies without anything for the ultimate healthy experience, but we probably would end up with no one in the family wanting to come to the table for meals anymore. Sometimes it is best to make the healthiest choice, but in a way that it can still be pleasing to the palate.

There is one thing that I say never needs be a part of your diet, and this will take a lot more willpower for your children than yourself. That is removing sugar and the common deserts from the diet at all times. We don't need these at all, and we have to retrain our brain when it tells us that we deserve this, and we have to have this. Sure, we really enjoy it and want it from time to time, but we don't need it. This may take longer to accept, and when we reintroduce foods back into your normal diet plan, this is one thing that does not need to come back in. Leave it out of your diet and leave it out of your house. Think instead of serving fruit for dessert. Or if you feel like you need something sweet, only serve desserts that have natural sweeteners in them. You can get enough extra sweets when you are out with friends or family and are confronted with the dessert after a meal; we don't need these in our homes, to be feasted on after each meal.

If this isn't possible to do, then consider the different recipes that are offered that have good ingredients we can have, and consume them instead.

As will be discussed later, sugar is our worst addiction and can cause us to raise the inflammation in our body, driving us to be much sicker and suffer from things we normally would not be affected by. There are so many good treats that can be made with honey or maple syrup that we can enjoy, and those have been broken down further so that we can process them naturally and so our body won't respond negatively to them overall. If one thing could be advised, that would be to pull all table sugar or any sugar-like substances out of your house for good and don't bring them back in ever, if possible. Just simply doing that will bring about the biggest change, and with time you will notice a big difference.

Once things have been going well and you seem to have a good handle on this lifestyle change and your family is handling it pretty well, what can you do when you reach the 90 days? There are two options you can consider, one being that you continue on as long as nobody is really complaining too much, and then you are fixed for life. The other option would be to introduce a few of the items back into your family's diet slowly, with the plan of bringing in 1-2 portions of grass-fed beef and pork per week out of the 21 meals. After week 1 of doing this, you can increase this to 3-4 times, but no more than 4 times a week. That would be beef and pork a total of 4 times, so you have 17 meals that are beef- and pork-free. When you do this, try to allow days in between to better process and digest the beef and pork since they are so complex in the diet. Once you have this down, you'll still be consuming more chicken, turkey, fish, and wild game as your majority meat source.

After the body adapts to this, then on week 3 you could bring in 1-2 portions of dairy, following the same format on week 4 with organic whole grains. It is best to keep these to a minimum of a couple times per month, or you will find that your family will be back with the same issues that you were wanting to eliminate from the beginning. When referencing the amount you can have of any of these things, it is suggested that you count one meal as one time per week. Some may have meals that have maybe both pasta and garlic bread, and you can consider that as one time. Remember the basics of removing these things, if you feel your family taking on more than these serving sizes. The key to becoming most successful is to bring back your lifestyle to these basics and consume as many vegetables as you want, with a smaller amount of fruit. Eat palm-sized portions of meat and grains, and no desert. Don't waste so much time measuring everything out, as it becomes cumbersome and time-consuming. Make it simple and do what is handy by using the palm of your hand to measure everything out for yourself.

The best way to start to improve a child's nutrition, or even a family's, in fact, is to take them back to basics. Eat the real food! Fruits and vegetables are the staple foods that should be found at every meal and for snacks in between. Eliminate all the processed foods with the extra additives and refined carbo-hydrates. You are what you eat, and if we feed the wrong types of bacteria to our gut microbiome, it negatively impacts our health and the health of our children.

Other great foods that can be good snacks or great sources of protein include lean meats, nuts, and seeds. "Lean meats" includes chicken, fish, turkey, and wild game, as they are not as complex and dense as red meats. Small amounts of red meats in our diets are sometimes necessary. But as a society, we get too much of it, and our children consume too much complex proteins that don't have the time to break down in their gastrointestinal tract before they consume another serving of it. Especially for those of us that live in the Midwest, where there is easy access to this source of meat. So then one would ask, "What is the real problem with eating too much beef or pork?" The problem is that it takes much longer for it to make its way through the digestive system and break down and be used in the body, so we eat 2-3 meals a day of these complex proteins and soon we have it sitting in our gut. Now, what happens to animal products that sit in the perfect temperature for a long enough period without moving on? Yes, you guessed it. It rots! This then is causing further damage to the gastrointestinal tract and leads to increased inflammation. Then we add a whole lot of other foods that increase inflammation, which include many of the grains, and of course, sugar.

Once we break down this gastrointestinal membrane, we start to lose the ability for good nutrients such as vitamins and minerals to be absorbed into the body as they slip through and pass out into our waste. This leaves many children with less-than-optimal health and deficient in nutrients that not only would heal them, but also drive sickness away. The other aspect that we need to look at is the point that the gastrointestinal tract has a direct connection with the brain through the vagus nerve. So, if the gut is inflamed, it has a direct impact on the brain. See how all this works together, and then we start to see our children not doing so well in school or acting out. This also goes along with those children that suffer with neurological deficits and have learning disabilities such as ADD, ADHD, OCD, etc. Cleaning up the diet and healing their gut can lead to a much stronger functioning brain and reduce many of the symptoms they may have.

So, start with the basics by removing any processed foods from the diet and increasing their vegetables to 2-3 more servings compared to fruit. Eat as organic as possible! I know this costs a lot more and not all families can support this. If that is the case for you, don't panic—do the best that you can, as it's more important that they get the vegetables in than to worry that they're all organic. Sugars have to be removed from the diet, as this is one of the leading aggravating factors to inflammation and will only drive it higher. We will talk about sugars more in a bit. This isn't something that will happen overnight, and the more enthusiastic and positive you can be with these changes, the more your children will see the importance and want to make a difference as well. Remember that it all takes time, and each day you make one step a little closer, the better you will be and the bigger the difference you will make in your children's life.

WE HAVE FOUND THAT HAVING A CONTAINER IN THE REFRIGERATOR WITH FRESH CUT RAW FRUITS AND VEGETABLES THAT CAN BE PULLED OUT AT ALL TIMES AND SNACKED ON MAKES IT AN EASY OPTION FOR THE KIDS TO HELP THEMSELVES TO A GOOD SNACK.

When it comes to snacks for children, this can be one of the most challenging changes to make. There aren't a lot of options, and it makes it difficult to find simple things that children would like to eat that would support proper growth and healing the gut. We have found that having a container in the refrigerator with fresh cut raw fruits and vegetables that can be pulled out at all times and snacked on makes it an easy option for the kids to help themselves to a good snack. The biggest concern with many snacks is that they contain such high levels of unhealthy sugars such as high fructose corn syrup. We are trying to eliminate this from the diet, so we don't want to bring it in for snack time. Plus, eating this type of snack in the middle of a school day will give them a fast and furious burst of energy and then they will crash quickly, about the time they are ready to learn.

It's true that most children won't automatically run up and say, "Oh Mom, I'm hungry! I want some of these good vegetables for my snack!" In fact, if we are honest, this may be one of the biggest struggles we will be faced with, and they will turn up their nose time and time again. Let me tell you that they will not starve to death, even if they like to imply this! If you set a container filled with a variety of vegetables and fruits on the counter or table where the kids can reach it when they are hungry, eventually they will eat some. They may pass it by several times, turning their nose up, but if you leave it there long enough, it will disappear!

When it comes to vegetables, as parents you don't need to limit their intake, as kids can eat as many as what their body can handle and take it. Obviously, if they clean the house out of food you may have to add some limitations, but I have yet to meet any family where all their children will do this. As was mentioned earlier, you can also add nuts and seeds in a bowl for a good snack to munch on. Something to just be mindful of is to keep peanuts to a minimum, as they have a higher content of the wrong fat and can cause more harm if consumed in large amounts. It truly can be as simple as this, and with a little practice these changes will happen, and you will be able to reflect back on how relatively easy it went.

Sugar is one of the most addictive foods that we all consume, which makes it the hardest to remove from our diet. But what damaging effects it has on the body, and especially on the behavior of our children! So many times, our children will eat a breakfast high in sugar content, such as cereal, and they will be bouncing off the walls as they begin their school day. Many times, we see increased behavioral issues with this and they will get into trouble and cause disturbances. About the time they start to settle down and the sugar burns off, it's about time for lunch. So, then we stuff them with more sugar over lunch and repeat the process.

THERE'S ENOUGH SUGAR IN A SIMPLE BREAKFAST OF CEREAL, MILK, AND A GLASS OF ORANGE JUICE TO FILL A HALF-PINT JELLY JAR.

Sugar drives inflammation through the roof and extinguishes the ability for the body's gut microbiome to properly heal. That's why you will see those children that consume higher levels of sugar suffer from colds and the flu more frequently than those that reduce it from their diet. We aren't talking about the natural sugars that can be found in fruit, but the artificial sugars that are found in so many processed foods and beverages. Those that were present at the Sprigs® Motherhood Conference were able to see how much sugar is contained in a single breakfast of cereal, milk, and a glass of orange juice. If one was to consume that in straight sugar, it would fill a half-pint jelly jar. When you multiply this throughout a child's day, you can see how fast that would add up. A 12oz can of pop fills half a jelly jar full of sugar, but what if they drink two cans? This has damaging effects on their body and gut, and often is so addictive that one cannot just stop without hard work and determination.

When children are already struggling neurologically, sugar alters their brain so much more that it can take days for them to recover and return to a somewhat normal brain function. Then they consume these levels day after day, and it's no wonder we have an increase in neurological deficits. I urge each family to strongly take a stand against sugar and use alternatives such as honey or maple syrup. Whole-leaf stevia can be used sparingly, but we don't know what long-term effects on the body this could have or if it can cause other damage. (NOTE: Please do not use raw honey on children under the age of 1, as this can cause damaging effects and cause them to build up allergies. But do children at that young age need sugar or sweetener anyway? Probably not.) When you start to use these natural sweetener replacements in all baking and daily use, it may take a little while to get used to it, but you will soon see a strong difference in how your family functions. It does take some time to get used to, but if you can adapt, it will help save you as parents from many hours working with your children either from being sick or hyper from a sugar high. God gave us the perfect sweeteners, so why not use them?

WHEN CHILDREN ARE ALREADY STRUGGLING NEUROLOGICALLY, SUGAR ALTERS THEIR BRAIN SO MUCH MORE THAT IT CAN TAKE DAYS FOR THEM TO RECOVER AND RETURN TO A SOMEWHAT NORMAL BRAIN FUNCTION.

This next topic isn't one that many want to talk about or even consider when it comes to nutritional support. We all know it's part of becoming healthy and know that we must do it in order to reach our goals. But it tends to be the first thing that gets let go at the end of the day, only making it to the "someday" list for most. Now, as a parent, you may think to yourself that your children get plenty of exercise each day. They are running around and playing hard, tormenting their siblings and probably adding those gray hairs daily to your head. But what we have to realize is that even if we eat perfectly, but just sit around on the couch and don't move much for the rest of our lives, we're not going to get the positive results that we could have by eating well and exercising.

We want this exercise to include around thirty minutes where they are doing a specific act of exercise. That could be riding their bike or walking/running continuously. Most of the time it can be very challenging for parents to work this into their busy schedule each day, and once again it gets put by the way. I ask that you please consider involving the entire family in this event. Right after dinner, or any good time throughout your day that seems fitting, gather everyone around in the living room and simply join together in doing something. It can be as simple as performing sit-ups, jump-ups, jumping jacks, or running up and down sets of stairs as a family. You can set up challenges in your house for everyone to join in and keep track of how many they do each time and record it. This then promotes a healthy reward at the end. This will drive them and encourage the whole house to get involved. Also, I challenge many of you to think outside the box when considering little trips for the family. Consider hiking or nature trails or simply taking a family bike ride on the weekend to help get everyone moving instead of just sitting in the living room.

It has been shown that trying to motivate one person to do a specific exercise task is near impossible, but getting into groups and encouraging each other can be very beneficial. The basic health benefits of this simple thirty minutes will take you and your children into the next level and support the longevity of your health. It aids in the mobility of digestion, allowing for food to be processed much better. It increases the blood flow to all areas of the body, especially to the brain, which can help improve the performance of your children in school. It aids in wound healing and helps fight off many of the common sicknesses. This is only the beginning of the list, but how we feel after exercising, along with reducing our fatigue and the draggy feeling our children have, will boost your energy overall. Exercise will also reduce the potential for disease and fight off obesity, which continues to steadily rise in the children of today. If you do feel that you need to make any nutritional changes in your child's life, simply incorporating this into their life could be the biggest impact you will notice lifelong. It's simple; start off slowly with five-minute increments and build from there, and soon you will reach the thirty-minute mark. This doesn't have to be done overnight, but one step at a time will begin the ultimate change to their health.

When it comes to working with food as our main source of survival, we often neglect the biggest source that makes up most of our body: Water! We as parents tend to consume more water than our children, but so often our children don't take in enough water either. The research varies as to how much water makes up our body mass, but we can say more than 75% of our body is made up of water. So, why do we forget about it so much when it has such an important role? We have no problem grabbing those soft drinks or juices for our children, but this isn't the pure water that their bodies need. A good rule of thumb that I like to express to all of my families is to have an idea of what your child weighs, then take their body weight and divide it in half, and this will give you the number of ounces they should be drinking each day. It doesn't have to be a complex mathematical equation. It can be simple, and then you can have a designated bottle or container so you always know if they were able to consume their water intake. This same bottle can go to school with them, and they can take it anywhere they need, but it's always present.

Water will re-hydrate the body so it functions like it should. But, most importantly, it aids in digestion, helping the children process the nutrients that they need. It also aids in flushing the bugs that they don't need or want out of their body, which prevents them from getting sick as often. Once again, water hydrates the powerhouse of the body, the brain, and provides the nutrients and minerals it needs as well. Our brain depends on lots of water intake. When we deplete this and run it low, it also will run less efficiently, resulting in brain fog, fatigue, memory loss, etc. Why not supply the body with the simplest form of fuel that it can count on to keep it going?

"Just because something says 'gluten-free' or
'all-natural' doesn't mean it's healthy."

- Jackie Warner

3

GRAINS/GLUTEN

Fad or Fact?

IT FEELS LIKE A great honor to be nicknamed "Pillsbury Doughboy" at a young age. Maybe you earned this title because you consumed as much bread or pasta as you could handle, any time you could. Some of you probably can't relate to eating that much grain-based foods, but what you can relate to is the point that when we remove these from our diet, we don't have anything else to eat–or so we think. Do we consume more than we might think at a meal or even in a given day? What do your children eat as part of their meal, and what really contains gluten? We have heard over and over that we are gluten sensitive or gluten intolerant, but what does that really mean? How can you remove the gluten in your diet and still enjoy eating from time to time?

The topic of gluten and grains seems to come up everywhere and has taken the trend lately as the main focus of many diets. The spread of information about food sensitivities, specifically focused on gluten sensitives, has led more and more people to strive toward becoming gluten free. This concept is one that is valuable and has merit, but there is one concept that seems to be skewed a little, leading people to think what they are doing is good. The list of gluten-free items seems to be getting longer and longer, and when it has that label applied to the side of a package, we feel we are limiting the gluten intake into our diet. The issue is, are we really doing this for the right reasons, and are we truly eliminating gluten from our diet completely? Gluten is predominately found in grains, and really hasn't been considered an issue until the past ten years or so. The problem with the grains we eat is that we have modified them so much to increase the yields and sprayed them with such strong chemicals that we have altered their make-up, making them less valuable in vitamins and nutrients and even harmful to our gut. Then, as part of the standard diet, we consume so many of them that we start to damage our gastrointestinal lining through an increase in inflammation. When we get the increase in inflammation in our gastrointestinal tract, we get an increase in pain, fatigue, suppressed immune system, brain fog, and simply feeling "yucky", as our children would put it.

> **THE PROBLEM WITH THE GRAINS WE EAT IS THAT WE HAVE MODIFIED THEM SO MUCH TO INCREASE THE YIELDS AND SPRAYED THEM WITH SUCH STRONG CHEMICALS THAT WE HAVE ALTERED THEIR MAKE-UP, MAKING THEM LESS VALUABLE IN VITAMINS AND NUTRIENTS AND EVEN HARMFUL TO OUR GUT.**

The issue with gluten is that it's in almost everything that we consume. One thing is for sure, you don't find gluten in fresh vegetables and fruits. It is found in grains such as wheat, corn, oats, rice, and many other grain-based foods. This is the glue that holds things together. When we consume our breads and processed foods, they stay nicely formed and ready to eat because gluten has held it all together, preventing it from crumbling apart. That is why, when using alternatives that don't contain gluten, you will find them much more flaky and crumbly, not having the consistency that we normally expect.

The key point that one needs is that we don't need to consume so much gluten, and it really could be eliminated completely from our diet. This is extremely hard to do, and many children won't buy into this concept. So when introducing this to the family, it can be very challenging for them to understand. Removing both sugar and gluten can seem like you are waging a war against your family, and it makes it very challenging to alter or change your lifestyle. If you follow through with these simple steps, however, you can help reduce your family's gluten intake and help the body properly digest it and absorb the good nutrients it needs without damaging and affecting the body.

An interesting fact about gluten is that it's found in many more items than people are aware of. In fact, it is in just about everything that we consume. Many people think that good substitutes for gluten/grains are rice or corn. Unfortunately, those would have the same or similar properties of the straight gluten found in wheat and should be avoided as well. Also, when we consume gluten, it has the potential to stay in our body for several months, still negatively affecting how we react to it. So, when someone tells you they are gluten free, they most likely are not, and it is encouraged not to say the same as well.

You may reduce or try to eliminate gluten in your diet, but even some ketchup has gluten in it. Even if you consume something that has gluten in it, it can stay in your system for a week to six months or longer. If you say that you are gluten free and you eat one thing, it can affect you for a long period of time, and you now have gluten in your system. I have said this over and over to people that keep saying they are completely gluten free. If that is the case, you must only be eating vegetables, fruits, raw nuts/seeds, and some organic grass-fed meats. This is essentially one of the only ways you can be truly gluten free. Stop saying you are gluten free when you know full well that gluten can be found in your diet from time to time in the rice flour or corn chips you are eating. The same can be said when you are told that you're gluten sensitive and you cannot consume the same foods as others. That has a slight possibility of being true, but it is mostly brought on by ourselves and what we do and eat.

We don't wake up one day and become gluten sensitive and suddenly have all of these problems. We over-utilize this "diagnosis," and, in the end, it is the bad choices we make that cause us to react the way we do. If you are having a possible reaction to gluten, there is a possibility that you are over-consuming it on a daily basis and the inflammation in your body is reacting, causing you to feel bloated and have stomach cramps. There is no doubt that this can be a problem, and if you reduce your gluten intake to a manageable amount, these symptoms can go away. Even in children that suffer from a gluten sensitivity, this could have been brought on by what the mother eats, consuming too much and passing it on to her child pre-birth. It can also happen at a young age. Ultimately, our children can become sensitive to gluten because they are eating too much of it and their body cannot process it or handle the amount that they are taking in on a daily basis.

Our bodies will react, trying to tell us that we have too much and we need to back off a little through the headaches, joint pain, tummy aches, bloating, and the other symptoms that occur. If you go and get tested for allergies, of course it will come up as a gluten sensitivity or intolerance. If we can back that off and start to heal the gut, we can reduce the inflammation. One should be able to handle a manageable amount of gluten each week and not suffer from it. We shouldn't have all the gluten sensitivities and intolerances that we have today, and when we do, it likely falls under celiac disease instead.

The condition of celiac disease is a serious condition that can affect the small intestine and is caused by eating foods high in gluten such as wheat, barley, and rye. Those that suffer from celiac will know that they have it and that it triggers bloating, flatulence, constipation or diarrhea, extreme fatigue, anemia, weight loss, and the biggest one, malabsorption. It damages the small intestinal lining, causing the good nutrients to not be absorbed into the bloodstream but to be sent on to the waste system.

Again, simple gluten sensitivity will not give you these symptoms, but can lead to celiac-like symptoms if we do not treat the sensitivity. Not everyone who calls their own condition "gluten sensitivity" has celiac, and those that have celiac know they have it. At the end of the day, recognize what the true symptoms are and simply step away from gluten, as it is damaging your gastrointestinal lining and driving up your inflammation in the body. If your gut is inflamed, then all the white blood cell fighters will come to the gut to rescue it, leaving the other areas in the body depleted and raising the rates of inflammation. That is why you have pain in other areas, along with the malabsorption of good nutrients, leaving you with pain, brain fog, fatigue, and many of the other symptoms. If you have celiac disease and you have it properly diagnosed, then treat it as such and remove all gluten permanently from your diet. If you do not have celiac disease, then stop saying you have a gluten sensitivity and acting like you have celiac. Instead, reduce your gluten consumption, lowering your chances of having symptoms that cause you discomfort. It is simple as that, and can work that simple if you treat it that way. If you raise the bar so high and say that you have a complex digestive issue as gluten sensitivity or intolerance, when it is really a chemical sensitivity, then you are misdiagnosing a problem that feeds into a FAD that is happening today.

The point needs to be brought out again that in a traditional American diet, we over consume wheat and gluten-infested foods on a daily basis. Think about this scenario as you eat your breakfast and consume several slices of toast with your eggs. Then at lunch, you and your family eat 2-3 slices of bread for your sandwiches, finishing the day off with bread or rolls with dinner. This can go for any foods high in gluten. As was mentioned, most of the foods we consume are higher in gluten. So it doesn't have to be the ones we mentioned here. We eat this type of diet over and over each day. We do this for seven days a week, increasing and decreasing a little here and there each day. But overall, we do this about every meal, 365 days of the year. What an overload on our system, as we cannot handle this much or even process it in our body. It builds up and ferments in our gut, causing deeply rooted issues which lead to inflammation. If we can drop our consumption down to an amount the body can handle, we can reduce and eliminate this so-called "gluten sensitivity" that we all are suffering from.

Here are the guidelines that can help you: If we can truly remove gluten from our diet completely without any cheating for a couple of months, letting our body heal and improving our absorption rate, which will help us get the good nutrients into our body, we can reduce the inflammation and feel amazing. Then, when we feel it has cleared out and we have our energy back and our brain functioning again, you can slowly bring it back in a 2-3-week process by adding 2-3 grains per week, maxing out at 4. Yes, I said per week, which means that this is per meal, not intake of items and preferably letting time pass in between to digest and process it all. Once this happens, then we can maintain at that level, having 2-4 organic grains in a 21-meal span. If you ever start to creep back up with your consumption, then bring it back down to no grains and start over. Use how you feel as you gauge and monitor, because it has been shown over and over when we remove the irritants from our body and let it heal, we should be able to bring them back in and eat them in a clean form at a healthy level.

"BEING HEALTHY AND FIT ISN'T A FAD OR A TREND. IT'S A LIFESTYLE."
UNKNOWN

This may seem a bit of extreme and go against what you have been told in the past, but carefully consider it and think about what is being presented. We never used to have an issue with processing wheat or any gluten. So why are we having so many issues today? The issue is that higher production and high chemical content, along with overconsumption, have taken a toll on the body and have driven our bodies to respond. If we can give our systems a break and calm the negative immune response that is driving up our pain and discomfort, we can maintain a good balance of gluten in our diet and do well with it. We don't have to live with the fact that we will be suffering from this condition for life and can't enjoy what we want from time to time. It all comes down to moderation and developing a true understanding that in a good healthy diet based on a good healthy lifestyle, we can consume things like gluten if we prepare the body for it ahead of time and reduce it to a moderate level.

CONTROL YOUR INTAKE AND YOU WILL SEE RESULTS BOTH YOUNG AND OLD; ABUSE YOUR INTAKE, AND YOU WILL SEE THE EFFECTS.

I compare this as well to consuming a good thing over and over and self-indulging over and over again. Consider this: If we consumed large amounts of cotton candy daily because we loved it so much, what would be the outcome? If you ask a child, of course they would say it's a "happy day, every day!" But as adults, we know without a doubt what the outcome may be, and we have to realize that gluten can do the same thing. Control your intake and you will see results both young and old; abuse your intake and you will see the effects.

If you are limiting the effects of gluten in your diet and trying to heal your family's tummy, consider removing all grains from your diet for a period of time. You need to set a time where this can be done, and I would suggest that you don't go over a 90-day period of elimination. Now, with that said, some will say, "I still need a little longer," or, "We struggled for a bit in the beginning," and that is okay. Each family is a little different, and how long it takes is up to each individual. It is mentioned not to go over a 90-day period of complete elimination of gluten because we all can grasp the idea that we can handle a 90-day period. We as humans need landmarks and know that unless we will die from something, we need an end date to something we really don't want to do. Even children understand this method and know that they can do something and watch the days go by knowing it will end. If you set a time period of 90 days, you have that end point and you can work toward it, often times realizing that 60 days in this is not too bad and you feel better about it as you go. You lose track of the 90 days and soon you may run into a longer period without realizing it, and it now has become the normal. If you choose to only do this for a week or two, it will be difficult to see actual changes, as the gluten won't have the time to be expelled from the body. We won't feel or see any changes, and that will give us the unfortunate will power to say, "This doesn't work." Of course it doesn't work, because we didn't allow enough time for it to work. Be realistic in all the goals you set when it comes to making the changes in your nutritional lifestyle. Create environments that are simple and ones you know you can achieve and build on your plan. Going for the worst task first makes it seem unobtainable and will only set you up for failure early on. When we fail early on, we won't have the push or desire to move forward. Setting up a plan to make even the tiny adjustments count will allow you to reach the bigger task much easier.

We have already discussed gluten, and even though gluten is a large field, there are other things you should avoid like wheat, barley, rye, rice, and corn. Anything that contains these substances either has direct gluten in them or has similar effects of gluten that will cause trouble in the body. Removing all of these during your healing process will promote a proper healing process. Just as if you cover a burn wound and make sure you stay away from the stove, if you keep your fingers close to the stove uncovered, you will keep aggravating and harming the area that is sensitive to the first burn. This is no different with our body, and we have to remove any form of gluten to actually heal. There are many theories out there that corn and rice are not the same and we often substitute gluten with these two ingredients, labeling them gluten free. This may be true, but they have the same effects as gluten, so why use them? There are other options that can be used, such as coconut flour, almond flour, spelt, sprouted grains, flax seed, cassava flour, quinoa flour, and several others. These take the gluten aspect out of it completely, and help you to still enjoy some of the family favorites and limit the exposure you have. Sure, the flavor isn't the same, but it does give options and gives you the opportunity to still have what your family loves and enjoys.

Look at the package and review what is inside of it before you just buy anything that is gluten free. They have slapped that label on everything, and it can be misleading. It appears to be more of a FAD now and not really a true realistic representation of why they would put that on there. They may use mainly ingredients that are free from wheat, but did they substitute it with corn? We have to carefully consider this if we are going to make this change and not get ourselves wrapped up in the gluten-free drive for healthier living.

WE HAVE TO CAREFULLY CONSIDER THIS IF WE ARE GOING TO MAKE THIS CHANGE AND NOT GET OURSELVES WRAPPED UP IN THE GLUTEN-FREE DRIVE FOR HEALTHIER LIVING.

If you want to reduce this intake, which you should do for a while, then go back to the complete basics of good vegetables and remove it. But stay away from labeling yourself gluten free. You are eating a healthy diet for a healthy lifestyle, and that is why you choose not to consume one thing or another. If you label your family gluten free, it will drive a separation from others in your family, making your kids establish a difference that they can recognize in themselves. They will turn away from what you are doing and not desire to be healthy, wanting to be normal instead. What we want is for them to establish a normal healthy lifestyle, not be identified with a specific label.

Just to run through the gluten area of control and how to proceed with our family: First, start to slowly remove all gluten from the diet. This can take several weeks to a month to completely remove it. Then, stay completely clear of it for 90 days to clean and repair your digestive system, noting how you feel and how the behavior of your children improves. Then at the end of 90 days, slowly start to bring it back in, keeping it to a maximum of 2-3 times per week for several weeks and then adding up to 6-8 times per week after that. There is no specific number, but implementing controls to the limit you can have each week will keep you consistent and limit how much you're willing to eat. If you find that some symptoms seem to come back, step back and consider whether your intake increased a bit and if you need to bring it back to the normal levels. It is strongly encouraged that you give this an honest try and see how you feel different when you bring these levels down. You may reduce your bloating or fatigue; you may have more energy than you did before. Or you may not feel anything, and you just know that you are doing the best that you can for your body. When we do this and make a conscious effort, we will be rewarded with long-term health for not only ourselves but for our family, and our families for many generations to come. We have to make that change because the food industry will not make it for us.

"Put away the notion that dairy is a health food. It is not!"

- Dr.Mark Hyman, MD

4

DAIRY

The double edge sword

THAT WAS A HARD discussion to have, to remove many if not most of the grains from your diet and try to maintain that for a period of 90 days with the entire family. But the amazing feeling you will have when you start to notice the difference in your children will be well worth it. As you digest that information, we need to take it a step further. Really, it doesn't matter which order you do these in; whether you reduce dairy or grains first, they both need to be removed from the diet. For some of you this may be more than you want to try, but dairy has caused a bigger intolerance than many of the other foods we can take in. If we were to put these into a list and categorize what we should take out and in what order, dairy should be within the top three. In fact, sugar should automatically be taken out, and right next to sugar would be dairy. There are enough that suffer from some form of lactose intolerance that it can almost be worse than grains to a point. Also, diary is found in so many things that it is hard to remove it completely, but going back to the simple foods like fruits and vegetables can make the difference and help you out.

When these concepts are explained to people, many times it is encouraged to be vegetarian and/or vegan. This is not true. This isn't a debate about whether a vegan or vegetarian diet is best. Both have their qualities and disadvantages. It wouldn't hurt at all to adapt elements of these lifestyles and bring them together as a strong, supportive healthy lifestyle. It has been shown that some strict vegetarians may suffer from lack of good essential nutrients found in some of the animal sources that they do not eat. However, when you pair their strong plant-based foods and a few animal sources, you have a good balance of essential nutrients. The vegan lifestyle eliminates all animal products from the diet providing you with a high level of nutrients that otherwise may not be found in your diet on a daily basis. But we need to realize that you can be misrepresenting the true vegan lifestyle and aren't aware of what nutrients you need to supplement that you'd normally get from the animal products you are taking out of your diet. Again, those that have very strong views on vegetarian or vegan dietary lifestyles know what and why they do what they do. This is only to bring a little awareness to those who want to pursue these lifestyles, make sure you do plenty of research to support why you are doing it and what you need to supplement to make sure your body is getting all the valuable nutrients it needs on a daily basis. It should be strongly mentioned that either of these

> THIS ISN'T A DEBATE ABOUT WHETHER A VEGAN OR VEGETARIAN DIET IS BEST. BOTH HAVE THEIR QUALITIES AND DISADVANTAGES. IT WOULDN'T HURT AT ALL TO ADAPT ELEMENTS OF THESE LIFESTYLES AND BRING THEM TOGETHER AS A STRONG SUPPORTIVE HEALTHY LIFESTYLE.

lifestyles can be supported with the proper knowledge and guidelines for you to follow.

There is always that little distraction that needs to be mentioned on the topic that we were trying to discuss, and that is how dairy has an effect on the gastrointestinal tract of an individual and causes them to be called "lactose intolerant." There is a difference that needs to be noted between dairy products and what truly causes the problem with dairy. Dairy has two components that can cause a digestive system to struggle a little and, in the end, drive up the immune response. Dairy contains lactose, which is the sugar portion of the dairy products. It is formed by two monosaccharides, one being glucose and the other being galactose, which then forms a disaccharide compound that we consume through many dairy products. The galactose is one monosaccride that our newborns need to get from breast milk if possible, as it enhances the nerve and brain development in our little ones. However, when we consume dairy, we end up with a disaccharide of both a glucose and galactose compound that cannot be broken down as easily in our digestive system. Some people do not have the strong enzymes needed in the body that get dumped into the digestive system to break down these disaccharides to produce the individual monosaccharides, which causes the body to recognize that there might be a foreign object in the body and it has to send a defense to it to protect the body. This subsequently brings up the immune response, since they are the ones that are coming to battle this foreign invader in the body. Once this happens, we get symptoms that present as lactose intolerance and bring down the overall performance of the gastrointestinal tract, leaving one to react with a tummy ache, earache, bloating, burping, and overall not feeling well at all. That is why those who suffer from this will reach for products that say lactose free, so they do not have to go through this process of the body's inability to break these down. The other alternative would be to take additional supplementation of enzymes to be able to break this down and produce the better environment for the digestive system to function. Either one can be helpful, and many that do this know it works. By reducing this reaction, they feel so much better and can live a relatively normal life.

Then we have the other side of the table, that dairy can attack our body and cause us more damage, which would be the protein side of things. The protein source in dairy is called casein, and is hard for our digestive system to process. The argument that can be made is that I am gluten free, but I still have a lot of symptoms that did not go away. Casein, the protein source in dairy, can react in the body similarly to gluten and can be over-consumed. This can be for those who are not lactose intolerant and can cause the same immune response in the digestive system, driving down the overall performance of the digestive system.

Even if you feel that you consume a good, healthy diet, but you are continuing to consume larger amount of dairy, you may suffer from an overload, which then affects you just like gluten will. The term, which has the same constituents as gluten, will tell you that it is not gluten, but it will react in the same way that gluten may react in the body. We have to treat it the same way and eliminate it from our diet.

Some may not know they are having trouble digesting dairy, but they have reached a point that they don't feel well and know that something has to change. Because of the popularity of gluten, we tend to remove it and then figure out that we are not completely better. So now what is the problem? People don't realize they got rid of one inflammation trigger but are still indulging on large amounts of dairy. Remove that dairy and you may see that it does help you feel better than you did before. It was mentioned before that dairy is found in a lot of cooking. So how can we get away from it completely? There are other alternatives such as coconut milk or almond milk that can be used and are good sources. Cheese is one of those things where substitutes are harder to find, so it is recommended that you eliminate it completely if you can. Now, there are sour cream, butter, and cream cheese that get brought up all the time, and you may wonder how you substitute with those. This is a little more challenging, unless you eliminate them completely and learn to eat things that do not have them in the diet at all. This can be done, but it can't be denied that it isn't easy. The easiest way to process this in a realistic way for your family is to think about how much you are putting into the recipe that you are making. Could you use a substitute for this recipe that wouldn't change the taste or the outcome very much? This can be a little

THE OTHER OPTION TO THINK ABOUT IS TO MAJORLY LIMIT YOUR DAIRY INTAKE AND ONLY USE SMALL AMOUNTS OF BUTTER OR CHEESE TO JUST ADD A LITTLE FLAVOR TO YOUR MEAL. IF YOU ARE ONLY USING SMALL AMOUNTS, BY THE TIME THIS HITS YOUR TUMMY, IT IS BROKEN DOWN TO A VERY MANAGEABLE AMOUNT, WHICH MOST OF THE TIME YOUR BODY CAN HANDLE AND PROCESS.

more time-consuming and not seem worth it. That is where a cookbook can be very handy (and you will find that resource at the end of this book). The other option to think about is to majorly limit your dairy intake and only use small amounts of butter or cheese to just add a little flavor to your meal. If you are only using small amounts, by the time this hits your tummy, it is broken down to a very manageable amount, which most of the time your body can handle and process. It's when we eat a pound of cheese and drink a glass of milk every single meal, along with the sour cream and cream cheese that are in our casseroles, that this will destroy our gastrointestinal lining and not allow us to process the nutrients we need. So, simplify your life and eliminate the main sources of dairy that you consume too much of, and get down to only those things that you put in the foods you make. Obviously, if you are lactose intolerant you must continue to do without those, because it still may affect you even in very small amounts. It could be urged that we need to work on the repair of our gastrointestinal tract, and we could possibly consume and process these nutrients better.

"HOW CAN YOU EXPECT YOUR BODY TO LAST FOR A LONG AND ENJOYABLE LIFETIME IF YOU DON'T PUT THE PROPER BUILDING BLOCKS IN THERE?"

DR. DAN ROGERS

The ideal situation would be to eliminate these negative dietary contributors from our diet, such as the heavy doses of dairy and gluten, and we would feel so much better. Just as was mentioned with the gluten, however, if we pull dairy out of our diet for a period of time and then bring it back in a moderate amount, that could still help our body to process it much easier. With dairy, if you can eliminate most of it completely that would be the best, because it has two components that can affect us as was mentioned—the casein and the lactose. The best option would be to take it away completely and have it only in special occasions or not at all. If you are a family that needs your dairy products, then reduce it over a 2-3-week period, trying to eliminate it completely from the diet. Once you have reduced it and taken it out of the normal diet, then go for 90 days trying not to ever consume any of it, just like with gluten. Once you have had that time to repair the gut, then you can slowly bring it back in the same way you would bring in the other products, consuming dairy only 1-2 times per week for several weeks, then taking it up to 3-5 times and maintain with that. The ideal would be never to reach the 5 times every single week and to alternate between dairy and non-dairy days to allow time for the gastrointestinal tract to process it all and get it through your system.

If you don't feel that you can do this with your family, especially if you are a family that includes big dairy eaters, then take those baby steps and consider making recipes that don't contain dairy. The cookbook referenced at the end of this book can be very helpful with that, as the work has been taken out already. Just like with gluten, if you begin to do this you will see noticeable changes in how you feel, and you may even see a change in your family when they aren't getting sick as much. What a huge relief if you could go several months without the runny noses or someone complaining about not feeling well. It can be done, as we have done this with our family and have seen huge results and reduced our trips to the doctor's office.

We all know that there are those weaknesses like lovely ice-cream that we just cannot get away from, but there are so many great alternatives. Why not try some of those out to see that you are able to make that change and still enjoy that great satisfaction after all? Lifestyle changes take time, and depending on what foods are important to you and your family, you can make the difference based on how well you can adapt these changes. It is necessary to remind all of us that healthy lifestyle changes don't happen overnight, just like the fact that you didn't get this way overnight. It all takes time and patience to reach the goal that you want with your family. However, with time, you will again see that the struggle you went through did pay off and you were able to reach the goal that you wanted, and your family is healthy and well now and into the future.

*"Sugar is **eight** times as addictive as cocaine"*

- Dr.Mark Hyman, MD

5

SUGAR

Cocaine?

IF THERE IS ONE thing that has gripped our world in daily cravings, it would be Mr. Sugar! Have you noticed that just about everything we consume nutritionally has some form of sugar or sweetener in it? Is it because we have to have it to live? Of course not! But when we are addicted to it, we must have it. It has been referenced in the past that sugar and high fructose corn syrup have the same addictive properties as cocaine. So, does that mean that we could be inhibiting our lives and the lives of our children by consuming too much sugar? I want to lay out the facts for you and then let you decide. There are plenty of options out there which we could substitute and make a healthier choice, but are we doing that?

We all have that sweet craving from time to time, and I understand that it's just not the same to grab an apple to munch on when the craving hits for a candy bar, or that our children would rather eat the Lucky Charms than eggs each morning before they head out the door. But one thing I want you to consider is: Why are we so sick in America today? Why are we suffering from obesity in our young people, with a much earlier onset of diabetes than ever before? Why do children not perform as well in school as they should, and why do we have this brain fog so early in the day?

Stop and consider that sugar is in everything that we eat, and the more that we eat, especially our children, the more we crave it. Sweeteners are added to almost everything found on the market today because they want us to crave it so we buy more. Look at carrots, for instance; they have natural sugar, but do you see children throwing a fit in the checkout lane at the grocery store because they want some carrots to munch on? Do our families reach for a second helping of dessert or for another spoonful of peas? These are all simple questions we need to be asking ourselves and evaluating our family's eating habits.

It doesn't take long before we can see that maybe you and your entire family are addicted to some form of sweeteners. Some of the common effects of sugar are obesity, brain fog, sickness, diabetes, etc. What does it do to our body, and why is it so bad for us? Poor sweeteners are the fuel to the fire of inflammation. They give a quick burst of energy and then it's gone. If we continue to consume more to be able to function on a regular basis, it still gives the energy bursts for us to function. But we then store the excess in the liver as glycogen. We continue to add to that excess over and over when we consume so much that we eventually overload the liver and reduce the function that it was designed for, purifying the blood. When the purification does not happen, we start to put stress on the entire cardiovascular system, which then makes our heart work harder than ever before. This can lead to premature plaque buildup around the heart and cause many of our children to have increased cholesterol issues, raising their risk of premature death.

Another fact is that we aren't regulating the glucose in the body through the liver, which in turn affects the pancreas, causing hormone and enzyme release to be overworked to compensate for the poor performance of the liver. When this happens, the pancreas stops functioning at optimal performance because it is being overworked, and it shuts done. When we lose the proper function of our liver and pancreas, we have full-blown diabetes, which continues to appear in children at an increasingly younger age. What we don't realize is that once they go on insulin, it takes away the need for the pancreas to make it and then the body thinks that it has no need for it, and the pancreas will never support itself again. Once this happens, we lose that function completely, which then puts more stress on the liver, causing it to purify the man-made insulin. The liver is not preforming optimally, and it will soon become inhibited, which will put pressure on the heart and kidneys, putting many of the people affected in renal failure at an early stage. Do you see how this compounds the problem and why we are struggling as a society over and over with increased healthcare issues and costs?

THE STANDARD AMERICAN DIET TENDS TO LEAD TO POOR GUT HEALTH AS IT BREAKS DOWN THE GASTROINTESTINAL LINING AND MAKES THE GUT LESS ABLE TO ABSORB THE GOOD NUTRIENTS, PASSING THEM INTO OUR WASTE SYSTEM.

Let's take another approach to this. What does this do to our gastrointestinal lining, since it has to pass through that before we can use it in the body? Sugar and processed sweeteners drive inflammation, which in turn drives sickness. As described before, it's like adding gasoline to an already flaming fire that will explode when you aren't paying attention. The standard American diet tends to lead to poor gut health as it breaks down the gastrointestinal lining and makes the gut less able to absorb the good nutrients, passing them into our waste system. The problem is that we don't support our gut and feed it the amount of healthy food it needs, so this happens day after day, which soon inflames our gut. Then, when we consume improper sweeteners, it drives the inflammation up. When our body is trying to repair the inflamed gastrointestinal lining and we are exposed to sickness, we cannot fight off the new sickness as well because our white blood cells are busy working to improve the health of our gut, leaving us sick for long periods of time. This is especially true for our children. They recover from some sickness, but their immune system is still trying to regain strength, and then they are hit again when they are exposed to the sickness of their fellow schoolmates. If we enhance their diet with lots of good vegetables, that could help in the healing of the gut and reducing all sugar that fuels the inflammation. We can then begin to heal and fight off sickness much more quickly. It is a complete cycle that keeps happening over and over again.

"THE AVERAGE CHILD NOW HAS NEARLY 20 TEASPOONS OF SUGAR DAILY—6 TIMES THE RECOMMENDED AMOUNT."

UNKNOWN

So, how can we reduce this intake and use the right sugars that can support the proper healing and nutrients for the body and brain? First remove and eliminate all refined white and brown sugar from the home. Get them completely out of the house and out of your family's life. That would be the first place to start, and then you can begin to replace it with natural forms of sugar such as honey, maple syrup, coconut sugar, and maple sugar. Remember that fruit has its own natural sugar, so you can always use that in the appropriate place as well.

It may take a while to reduce our sweet tooth, as it is often said that not all baking tastes the same with these other sweeteners. I understand this, but we have also damaged our palates and brains to think we need sweets, so it takes time to adapt to foods that taste less sweet and have a slightly different texture. We do have a new cookbook that just came out with recipes, with these sweetener substitutions in them already. Please contact us if you would be interested in purchasing one. Some may not be satisfied with these sweetener choices, and better choices than regular sugar would be pure stevia, xylitol, or erythritol. These aren't as high on the recommendation list because they are sugar alcohols and can cause other issues like nausea, bloating, upset stomach, and diarrhea if used in large amounts or for extended periods of time. It is also hard to find plain organic stevia with no additives, which are used to hide the bitter aftertaste. Long-term use of the xylitol, erythritol, or stevia could lead to less effective liver function and buildup of toxins in the body if used for years. If they are used with discretion they may be okay, but the natural sweeteners are always the best as they are broken down and in the simplest form that is easily digested by our body. There is mixed research demonstrating that stevia, xylitol, and erythritol have both positive and negative long-term effects, which leaves it inconclusive as to whether it's really safe to expose our children to them for long-term use.

The last topic that comes up is about the glycemic index and how foods affect the blood sugar levels in the body. Let's face the fact that if you heal your body through proper nutrition and reduce the inflammation in the body, you should be able to handle the multiple levels of glycemic index without huge in fluctuation in your blood sugar levels. So how do you control the glycemic index in your daily food intake the easy way? Consume mainly vegetables, especially those green leafy vegetables, and eliminate processed or prepared foods and sugar. This will begin to balance out your blood sugar levels so when you eat fruit or those carbohydrates that have a tendency to increase your glycemic index, they can be balanced out by the high support of the vegetables you are consuming. It's an easy process and method to follow; consume mainly vegetables with a little fruit, adding in lean meats, and your daily diet is one that would solidly support a healthy lifestyle and keep everything in check.

> **"YOUR BODY DOESN'T HAVE THE ABILITY TO TURN GARBAGE INTO A HIGH QUALITY PRODUCT. ALL OF YOUR CELLS, MUSCLES, SKIN, BONES, ETC, ARE BUILT BY THE FOOD THAT YOU SUPPLY. CHOOSE WISELY."**
>
> UNKNOWN

We can travel from doctor to doctor to resolve all kinds of issues and read book after book to figure out why our children are doing what they are doing. But when you reflect on what they are eating and their daily activity, are we providing them with everything we can to help naturally heal their body? It's not always an easy road to change your entire household's eating and cooking habits, but it has to start somewhere, and making those little changes one step at a time can begin to make those bigger changes. Just think—if you could eliminate one cold or flu spell by simply changing what your child eats, how effective could this be? Not to mention, they are headed on a lifestyle change that could affect their entire life, even into adulthood. If you feel you aren't ready to make this change right now, consider adding more vegetables to your family's intake each day and see how it builds from there. Remember, we have a cookbook that can help you cook healthier for the entire family, and all you have to do is contact us and order one to help ease that burden of trying to figure it all out alone.

*"If it's made in the garden then I eat it. If it's
made in the lab then it takes a lab to digest."*

- Kris Carr

6

MEAT

A staple in the traditional diet....Needed?

PROTEIN...MEAT...these words usually mean one and the same in most households, and even a young child in America today would tell you that meat needs to be a staple of any meal of the day. We have been taught to think we can't sit down to one meal without having a good source of meat on the table to indulge in. Who can resist sitting down to a meal with the smells of a freshly grilled steak wafting through the air? In fact, I often hear that mothers and wives will say that their husband or sons would die if they did not have meat and potatoes for every meal. I want to challenge this thought process a little and help each one of you think a little beyond the meat and potato concept, hoping to slowly give you a glimpse into what can be done to change around the standard American diet and improve our health overall.

The average American today consumes way too much meat protein. The idea that we need protein, protein, and more protein to survive has been pounded into us. Each person (child or adult) only needs about 20-50 grams of protein per day. For every four ounces of beef, there are about thirty grams of protein, and who only eats four ounces of beef per day? Many will disagree with this thought process of too much meat protein, but as you read, consider what you might be doing to your body as you chew on that tender piece of meat at your next meal.

I've talked about this in the past, but the sickness of America today continues to grow rapidly and is affecting our children at an even higher rate each day. We have to stop and consider some of the facts that we are being presented with and ask ourselves, are we doing what we can to improve our situation? Do we need all of this meat, or essentially protein, that we consume on a daily basis? Will our children die if they don't have meat at every meal? We do need some protein in our life to help give us that higher level of energy to be able to function, aid our brain, and regulate our blood sugar levels. So, we need some protein in our daily life, and there is no question about that. But do we need as much as we think? What about all of the other sources of protein that we get from our diet? Consider vegetables. Have you ever heard of anyone telling you that you need to cut back on vegetables daily? Never! Some of the basic vegetables that we should be consuming daily have up to eight grams of protein per cup! If you were to encourage your family to increase their daily vegetable eating by 2-3 cups per meal, you would essentially receive

> **THE AVERAGE AMERICAN TODAY CONSUMES WAY TOO MUCH MEAT PROTEIN. THE IDEA THAT WE NEED PROTEIN, PROTEIN, AND MORE PROTEIN TO SURVIVE HAS BEEN POUNDED INTO US. EACH PERSON (CHILD OR ADULT) ONLY NEEDS ABOUT 20–50 GRAMS OF PROTEIN A DAY.**

up to 24 grams of protein per meal just from veggies! Do you really need all that meat when you have so many great benefits from good vegetables?

MEAT HAS GOOD QUALITIES, AS IT DOES PROVIDE COLLAGEN AND MANY OTHER GOOD BENEFITS. WE JUST DON'T NEED THE AMOUNT OF MEAT WE CONSUME DAILY, AND THE QUALITY OF MEAT SHOULD BE SELECTIVE.

I know many of you who are reading this would say that your family will never consume that many vegetables each day. I understand this, and most families today don't even come close to the proper amount of vegetables we need per meal; instead, they are being left out of the diet completely. This is robbing their body of the antioxidants and phytonutrients that are needed so badly to be able to fight off sickness and infection. This leaves our families battling sickness and at increased risk needing higher levels of medication. We know that we can naturally limit extra medication and help improve the overall health of our children with a few simple changes. Does this mean that they will never get sick again? Not at all! But it does reduce the likelihood that they may become sick, and helps them fight many of the common diseases such as early childhood obesity and diabetes.

Now that you are hopefully starting to understand that you need to increase the vegetable consumption in your life and the life of your family, please understand that you cannot accomplish this overnight. Do this in little steps, building as you go, meal by meal, and slowly you will begin to have noticeable changes that can be very rewarding in the end.

Meat has good qualities, as it does provide collagen and many other good benefits. We just don't need the amount of meat we consume daily, and the quality of meat should be selective. But consuming too much meat protein may be harmful also. Why? It can cause kidney disease, obesity, increased cholesterol, and more. Traditionally, most consume beef or pork as their main protein source. These two meats are more complex in nature, and their biochemical makeup is hard on our digestive system. Their complexity, along with being grown commercially, increases the accumulated antibiotics, hormones, herbicides, and pesticides that are a burden to our metabolism and are best to be avoided altogether.

"TAKE CARE OF YOUR BODY. IT'S THE ONLY PLACE YOU HAVE TO LIVE IN."

JIM ROHN

When you compare this to chicken, turkey, fish or any of your leaner meats, you will see that they can be broken down much more quickly. If we don't break down the complex proteins found in beef or pork, they tend to stay in our gastrointestinal lining for longer periods of time, and then they become inflamed and cause damage to your gastrointestinal lining. When it is inflamed, your gut doesn't allow the absorption of good nutrients to happen, and these essential nutrients eventually become depleted in the body. This then increases our risk of becoming sick because we don't have the vitamins and minerals needed to fight off simple illnesses. The body is working so hard against the inflammation in the gut that it doesn't have the resources to be able to fight off the bacteria and viruses we come in contact with. This problem is compounded even more when large amounts of beef and pork are consumed on a daily basis, and we don't allow our gut to reduce its inflammation and heal itself. If our gastrointestinal tract doesn't heal, it starts to affect our brain, as there is a direct connection between the gut and brain.

How can we fix this problem and decrease the risk of our gastrointestinal tract from becoming destroyed? Eliminate all the issues that are compromising it in the first place. Some of these we discussed in previous issues, but the one that is our focus would be the meat that we consume. Reduce your intake of beef and pork to only a couple of times a week. If you can get grass-fed beef, that is much better, as it does not have the toxic load and offers a healthier ratio of omega-6 and omega-3 fatty acids that are missing in the standard American diet. If you don't have access to this pasture-raised meat, do your best with your purchases and reduce your intake of meat, allowing extra time between the meals you have for it to process and get out of your body. You can replace this with lean meats (chicken, turkey, and fish) which can be broken down and utilized by the body much more quickly without having damaging effects. Even having a day where you don't consume meat but just vegetables can be helpful. If you do consume those meats that are non-organic/non-grass fed and are at a higher risk, consider including a good pre-probiotic in your daily supplemental regime. This will drastically aid in increasing the good bacteria in the gut, allowing you to reduce the ill side effects.

Hopefully you can use this as a guide to reduce the amount of meat you consume and increase the vegetables you need in order to help your body run more efficiently and safely for longer periods of time. Even the ability to reduce the risk of illness in our young ones could be a big step in the right direction. Consider the damage it may cause and slowly make that transition of healthier living for the entire family.

*"Sleep is the golden chain that
ties health and our bodies together."*

- Thomas Dekker

7

SLEEP

But I'm not tired!

SLEEP IS ONE OF the things that many of us wish we could get more of. This is something we dream our children would do just a little longer, or nap just a few more minutes longer. Have you ever found yourself groggy, hesitant to rise in the morning and start your day? Have you ever dreamed of sleeping all day, having the ability to just rest and relax? What if you could have this? What if you could get your children to have that restful night of sleep and always wake up feeling well-rested? Sleep isn't valued by today's young people, nor do most people realize the role it plays in our health. We do have the ability to reach our full wellness potential by taking some basic steps to improve sleeping patterns so we can wake up well-rested and ready to jumpstart our day. Making a few changes in your family's lifestyle can be well worth the rewards of good health.

Society isn't sleeping well today because of a whole host of reasons. You have your own set of reasons for why you don't wake up rested or feel like you are waking up multiple times during the night. Are you even able to fall asleep at night when you lay your head on the pillow, or are you laying there for long periods of time, letting your mind race with the many tasks you have at hand? What about our children—how are they sleeping, and why are they waking up so behind in the morning, needing to be dragged out of bed by their toes? It seems that they shouldn't have the cares of life bogging them down and keeping them awake or feeling unrested in the morning. Let's not limit the discussion to night—are you pounding down coffee or a Coke all day long just to make it through? Are you making it just past lunch, and then wanting to curl up and take a nap, unable to focus on what you need to do? Do you walk into your child's bedroom or notice they have crashed on the couch in the middle of the day? What about their schoolwork? Do you find that their teacher is constantly complaining that they seem checked out and not focused throughout the day? These are only a few examples of what many of us could be faced with daily.

The first step in achieving the proper sleep you need each night is to establish how many hours you need. The range of sleep time varies for an adult, a growing teenager, and a younger child. An adult should get an average of eight hours of sleep each night. Teens down to school-aged children need a little more sleep, about 8-12 hours per night. Dropping down to younger children, an acceptable range is around 12-14 hours per night. Then you have all the way down to an infant or newborn, who needs as much as 15-17 hours per 24-hour period. We can learn a lot from newborns and infants on sleep, as they get the required sleep that they need. Think about it—we don't tell babies to go to bed, they seek the sleep they need when they are ready. Now, common sense tells us that we cannot just curl up when we get tired and go to sleep in the middle of the day.

But we need to teach our body to get more sleep than what is the norm of today's society.

The all-time important question is: How can we get the sleep we need or get our children to get the sleep they need? We think we don't have the time to go to bed early or sleep for that many hours. It can be very difficult, and there are sometimes situations in our life that may allow us to get only a few hours each night. I can personally relate, as there was a time when I was only getting a couple of hours of sleep each night. But it takes a toll on the body, and soon we find ourselves in bigger trouble because our body starts to demand more sleep than we have time for. Our organs begin to shut down or become ineffective, and the body has to work that much harder in order to properly operate robbing even more of our needed energy to function daily. That's why so many of us start to run out of steam in the middle of the day, as we have maximized the energy that we had and have to depend on our stores to get us through. This leaves many adults and teenagers with brain fog and lack of motivation, making it harder to get up in the morning, increasing low self-esteem, depression, anxiety, sugar-handling issues, and a whole host of diseases and conditions that could have been avoided simply if we went to bed at a time our body needed to properly function.

We may have learned from a young age that we must go to bed at an early time, but very few of us accomplish what we set out to do. We can achieve getting our children down to bed in a timely manner, but then when it comes to us parents and older children, we seem to let time slip away by allowing ourselves to enjoy a few moments of getting some last-minute things done and relaxing before crawling into bed ourselves. By this point it could be very close to midnight, with the morning alarm ringing only hours away. Now let's face it that this may not happen every single day. But within a week or two, it can start to compound, adding to mental fatigue and reduced bodily functions. Then you compound the problem year after year, and we can quickly see how it may alter our organs and body systems to where they don't function at ultimate capacity.

SLEEP HAS JUST AS IMPORTANT OF A TASK WITH OUR BODY'S FUNCTION AND WELLNESS AS EATING RIGHT DOES.

I want to look at another approach, which would consider the body systems and how they can be altered through our sleep cycles. We have a circadian rhythm or sleeping pattern that we go through each night. This will take us through the different sleep cycles and help us go from a light sleep to a deep, dreamy sleep throughout the night. When we don't get to bed at a reasonable time, we alter this circadian rhythm, not allowing our body to properly go through all cycles of sleep which causes our brain not to rest. Also, when we rest, we better digest and utilize the nutrients that we took in throughout the day. This is done through our parasympathetic nervous system, and we need this time to properly pull all the vitamins and minerals out of our food as well. When we alter this, we decrease the clarity of our brain which then alters the directions it can give the body systems, especially our gastrointestinal tract. This then reduces the gastrointestinal tract's ability to properly function and digest food. When we can't break all of the food down, it essentially rots in our gastrointestinal tract, breaking down the walls and causing an increase in inflammation in our digestive tract. This all happens over and over, not allowing our bodies to properly digest the food that we need and pull the good nutrients out of our body.

Sleep is just as important for our body's function and wellness as healthy eating. I strongly urge you to focus on how you can improve your sleep in order to thrive above just being able to function on a daily basis.

If you begin now setting up your family's sleep habits, it will become a "normal" sleep cycle for you. If you don't begin now, you will never find the time or the drive to make it a habit in your life. If we don't change our current habits, they are only considered bad habits. But if we make a habit into a new normal, we create a lifestyle change which can be easily embraced for the rest of our life. If we don't continuously make a conscious effort to instill these practices into our daily lives, we continue down the path of self-destruction. This goes for everything that we do, but as an example, we can look at dieting. How many times have we dieted and lost the weight but then gained it back? Only to do this over and over every couple of months. The worst part is, we eventually accept where our body is and never really appreciate where we could have been. Then this gets instilled into our kids, they follow the same pattern that we do, and the cycle repeats. To prove this, simply look at all of the fad diets that are out there today. We wouldn't need those if people made a lifestyle change instead of dieting. This will be discussed in other areas of the book, but if you don't take anything else away from this, you need to know that you must change your life, not just implement a change for a period of time only to fall back into old habits—ones that will be inherited by our children instead of the healthy ones.

In order to begin this new normal, we must set a specific times to get to bed and wake up each day. This should include approximately eight hours of sleep each night. I know, I can already hear people telling me that they cannot get eight hours of sleep each night as they don't have time, or their kids won't go to sleep, or whatever the case might be. The excuses out there are abundant and there are plenty of my own that I could share. But what do we really want in our life? Do you want to have a healthy life for your children and grandchildren, or would you prefer to enter into a state of illness and decreased function, especially with the possibility of depleting the proper neurological functions and increasing our risk for brain death, leading to early onset of dementia and Alzheimer's?

Does lack of sleep predispose you to these early onsets? Not necessarily, but it can increase the possible risk and enhance them. Who would voluntarily sign up for something like that? So, to preserve our brain, body, and wellbeing, we need to establish a healthy rhythm of going to bed for eight hours a night. It is advised to set a specific time each night that is relatively normal (such as 9-10pm each night) and consistently abide by it. I know there will be times, such as the weekends, when you will have things going on but you can have overall consistency.

Once you have this established, you can move more into the pre- and post-bedtime preparations that will enhance your ability to go to bed. This should include not eating past 8pm each night, allowing your body to digest what it has in it and starting to slow the brain down for rest. If we are eating and fall into bed, our brain is ready to do work to process and utilize the energy that we just put into it. This will drive your energy levels up, reducing the ability to fall asleep or to fall into a restful sleep by keeping you awake much longer. Make it a habit to try to stop eating by 8pm, or at least two hours before you crawl into bed at night to allow it to process through the stomach and get into the digested state before you rest. This should be the same for children as well. I support that they can maybe have a healthy snack, but let's get that into their tummies two hours before they go to sleep. This will help them be much more calm when they go to sleep instead of being wired before they crawl into bed.

"THE MINUTE ANYONE'S GETTING ANXIOUS I SAY, 'YOU MUST EAT AND YOU MUST SLEEP.' THEY'RE THE TWO VITAL ELEMENTS FOR A HEALTHY LIFE."
FRANCESCA ANNIS

This can be hard, as we are sometimes out and about, but a good practice of this can be very beneficial if you try your best to take healthy snacks with you. We don't have to make this a production, just simply a process that we get used to. Each family will find their own way to make this happen and provide a simplified version of this. My most important goal is to create ways to be simple in an already complex world. If we create a simple path, we can maintain what we really want, and it reduces the risk of giving up in the end.

There is another thought I want to get out there to improve the functionality of a good night's sleep and enhance our alertness in the morning, making us ready to face the day. For some of you, this will not be a big issue. But for others, it is a struggle both young and old. One of the main issues is technology and screentime from a phone, tablet, computer screen, television, and everything in between. We are in an ever-advancing world where many cannot dodge the need for some of these devices and depend on them on a daily basis. We have to control and eliminate these from our daily use as much as possible, but most of all at night prior to going to bed. The research will show over and over that the light emitted from these devices will stimulate the brain and keep one's mind going for several hours after they put them down and try to fall asleep. This can be up to two or more hours before your mind can actually rest and begin its sleep cycle. So, think about it a little bit—when we go to bed late, and the last hour we are messing on our phones or devices of any sort and stimulating our brains, when do you actually fall asleep?

"EAT HEALTHY, SLEEP WELL, BREATHE DEEPLY, ENJOY LIFE."
UNKNOWN

I would challenge each one of you to put this to the test as I have done myself, along with many others that I come into contact with, challenging them to put down the devices 3-4 hours before they go to sleep at night. Every single one of them have determined that they have fallen into a deeper sleep and felt much more rested when they woke up the next day. I think you will find the same thing. This is because blue light stimulates the brain causing it to fall into an activated state of rest, and keeping the body in activated motion throughout the night causing restless sleep and making each person rise more fatigued than they went to bed.

Think about our children a little bit and what devices do to their minds before they go to bed, and how this can deplete their rest as well. We may feel that we function on less sleep. But what do they have to handle when they go to school and have to think critically? It doesn't happen, as so many of them need that extra sleep and their brains are so fatigued that they can't think on their own. We have a serious epidemic right now, as so many kids are on a device at a younger age than before and have no skills to be able to think on their own. This will be addressed more in a further chapter as well, but I want you to think about this for your children and those you come into contact with who might be experiencing it.

Exercise can play such a huge role in your overall sleep habits, too. Even though it's recommended to start your day by getting the blood flowing to help wake you up, this seldom seems to be the case. What about doing it after work, before you go to bed at night? This doesn't have to be a gym membership, and I will talk about this more in the exercise section. But most of this can be done right from your home, and often can involve the entire family. Again, it needs to be stressed that you do this several hours before you or your children go to bed in order to calm the body down. Again, this has been beneficial in helping many minds and bodies release some of the toxins and stresses throughout the day and increasing blood levels to the brain, causing oxygen-rich blood to fulfill the body's demands and reduce the risk of fitful sleep at night. It also can help enhance the body's organs and fulfill the digestive motion and organ functions quicker to sustain a well-balanced body for a longer time. I've even recommended to some that they do a quick 5-minute, fast run in place to stimulate the restful mind for sleep. This does not work for everyone, so further evaluation needs to be done before this is put into effect. This can be done in the morning or at night in order to be effective, and works well depending on the individual's needs.

As we drift off to sleep, this should give you some things to think about and prepare your mind for the upcoming days. I want to break this down into simple guidelines that you can begin to implement today to get results for yourself as a parent, but also to implement for your children. What if you could go get your children up, and they were already up and ready to go each day without prompting or dragging them out of bed? Maybe they are getting enough sleep so they can function on a regular basis without the mid-afternoon snooze. You can feel the joy of crawling into bed knowing that you have completed a day's tasks, but not overly exhausted that you don't recall your head hitting the pillow.

Remember to establish a good routine of going to bed at a decent time, set a specific time between 9-10pm each night and wake up at a specific time each morning. You might have to alter this if your schedule doesn't permit you to fall into this. These are sample times, but it should be something close to this on a regular basis. Don't eat or allow your kids to eat after 8pm each night. Get plenty of exercise, and it can also be helpful to get exercise a couple of hours before you go to sleep at night. If possible, do not try to squeeze an exercise in and then go right to sleep after. Put devices away, preferably no later than 8pm (but I would like to see this sooner as it will enhance your family life and brain function). Eating right, drinking plenty of water, and making time for good relaxation can also play a great role in how you will fall asleep. At the end, practice deep breathing and let your body relax by thinking on the blessings you've had each day. Then see how you will rise in the morning, feeling rested and able to tackle any task set before you.

There will be times that you won't get to sleep the length of time you want, or be able to go to bed at the time you want. The same will be said for your children, but the consistency of a solid routine is a value that many of us let slip away. We know how we feel if we don't get enough sleep, and we stumble out of bed grabbing for our coffee. What about the children? How will they be affected, and what is their body and brain going through when they lose even one hour of sleep each night? The focus doesn't need to be on legalizing a specific bedtime, as this then raises awareness in their head (and even in our own mind) that if we do not, we are breaking some forbidden rule or destroying our family, and that can induce a sense of destruction for our well-being also. Help them understand how much better they'll feel when they go to school and how they can retain information, or even be able to follow directions better at home and at school when they are well rested.

If we instill in our family a value that they should want to go to bed because they want to rest and allow their minds to slow down and relax, opening the possibility of dreaming, it can lead to a better feeling overall in the body. If our brain isn't functioning properly, then our heart may have to work hard, and our lungs have to make an even greater exchange of oxygen and carbon dioxide, leaving us to feel more tired. If we can help our brains to better process information and fight the stress we put on it, we will be able to overcome the deficits we have on our organs and body as a whole.

One game we play sometimes with our younger children is to see who can fall asleep the fastest. It's fun to challenge them, as they think they can beat me. However, in the end, I end up passing out before they do. When we wake up in the morning, they are eager to find out who won. Set goals and points if this seems to be a hard concept for your children to grasp and make them aware that the winner will be rewarded. Obviously this does not become as effective with the older ones, but simply asking them to go to bed for their sakes and helping them feel the difference is the best approach for their well-being. It may take some time for those older ones, but it will come into play especially if they can realize that on the weekend, they can take a break and stay awake a little longer. Remember, we all like a little reward for the effort we put in, even if we are a little older and should know better. Giving this a little bit of a trial and sticking with a plan does not make your teenagers babies, but guides them for their future. We want to do all we can for our children, and if we can provide them with easy-to-follow guides, they will in turn pass that on to their children.

Adding essential oil diffusers in each room and providing each member of the family with a roller bottle with calming oils to use each night can go a long way in helping everyone to get a deep and restful night's sleep. This in turn can help heal our gut and balance the body's microbiome, creating wellness all around.

*"Push harder than yesterday if
you want a different tomorrow."*

- Fabletics

*"Food is the most widely abused anti-anxiety
drug in America, and exercise is the most potent
yet underutilized antidepressant."*

- Bill Phillips

8

EXERCISE

That awful "E" word.

THE TERM "EXERCISE" creates so much anxiety in
people, causing many families to push it to the back of their
minds because they feel they are already getting enough each day.
So often there is such a misconception that goes along with this
that we don't do it at all, and we find ourselves in the same daily
routine without getting our heart rate up or that of our children.

There is so much value that can attributed to good proper daily
exercise that it needs to once again become a habit or lifestyle
that we participate in, and all ages need to be a part of this. As
we reflect on the statistics that were presented at the beginning,
it is troubling to see how the disease rate continues to go up,
especially those of our children that are affected with obesity

and childhood diseases. We have to step up and recognize how exercise plays a large role in our overall health, and what we do to continue the legacy is up to parents and how they work with their children to make sure they get moving.

Do we really know how much physical activity our children are getting in their daily lives? Although we shouldn't be inhibiting a little rest and quiet time is nice, we need to promote more exercise and physical activity in their daily lives. We are living in a society where exercise has become less and less common, and current technology is overtaking the minds and bodies of our children. We often feel that if they are going to school, they are very active and they get what they need throughout the day. That is not the case, and right along with proper eating, we have to work on physical activity with our children.

They may not be overweight or you may feel that they don't need to get out and play as much as they do, but research has shown that children starting from a young age should have about sixty minutes of vigorous activity each day for numerous health reasons including maintaining good bone development, increasing stamina and agility, and reducing obesity and diabetes. It isn't abuse or lack of love on your part as a parent to get them out and moving—this is taking good care of them, ensuring their body is functioning properly and giving them all they need to stimulate physical growth and development.

When we talk about exercise, this isn't saying that they have to lift heavy weights or spend hours in the gym. Many of us might think those that do this are the elite of the elite, and may want that look. However, this can be very dangerous for teens and younger children. As their bodies are developing, such forms of exercise can close off their growth plates and damage the ability for their bones to grow properly. This will lead to earlier stages of arthritis, and they may go through growing pains in the future that won't allow them to grow properly as they get a little older. This can also damage their spine, which can lead to back pain and dysfunction as they get into their adult life, leaving them on disability or down to a minimal workload. We don't want to push our kids to this level, but we do want them to be able to increase their heart rate and get the blood flowing throughout their body, thereby increasing the amount of oxygen in their body. This will also help bone development with increased red blood cell production and utilize the pushing action of the lymph system to move blood throughout the body.

The lymphatic system does not have a pump system to help move the excess fluids and toxins out of the body; we must utilize the movement of the body to help get the fluid into the lymph vessels. They are then squeezed by our muscular system to move back to the heart. This is how we can get the fluid movement throughout the body and get the bad toxins out of the system so they don't harm us. We also need to increase our lung compacity so that we can expel that stagnant air in our lungs and get good, fresh air back into our lungs for proper circulation and respiration. Not having that proper gas exchange in our body will lead to toxification through carbon dioxide, limiting our ability for our blood to become refreshed and utilized to the fullest potential. This will in turn reduce the function of the organs that need it, especially the brain, and drive down our executive function in the brain, leaving us with slower reaction times and imbalanced hormones. We have to get the air pushed out of our lungs, filling it with good air so the body can function and run properly. This doesn't mean a two-minute run, as that isn't enough to make that exchange and fully help the body do its job.

We first have to beat the odds that we aren't doing this because we have to. We are doing this because we want to improve our overall health and longevity and enhance our body's function to properly digest and improve blood flow and to increase our brain function. It is your investment to your health and life. Just as many of us have tried to prepare ourselves for retirement, what if you did the same for your body? The same can be said for our children today; we need to help them learn that they need to invest into their lifelong change in improving their health and wellness. This doesn't have to be the forbidden task or the one that you keep putting off for another day. It must be one of the top priorities that we take part in each day and involve our children in the same. It doesn't have to be a complex, hour-long workout to be successful; it can be done right in your home and involve the entire family.

Today much more of our work is automated, so we have much less physical labor and a lot more time to sit on the couch. You can deny this all you want and say that you have implemented set times in your family's daily activities. But at the end of the day, exercise is not part of many family's lives, even on the weekends. Let's make this investment and start moving to enhance the function of the body and mind of our children and ourselves.

There are so many gym memberships out there that would truly promote the proper exercise that is needed. Many of them have personal trainers or group trainers that can help those who want to reach their exercise and wellness goals while giving much-needed support. However, these gym memberships take lots of commitment, planning, time, and lots of money, especially for a family to be able to support going on a continued basis. Then the scenario that often plays out is that a person or family may be committed for the first month or two and then they quit because it is too much to keep up with. This happens to so many people that it soon becomes the norm, and this is why you will see gyms running specials for the introductory months just to try to keep business going.

WE CAN TALK ABOUT NUTRITION ALL DAY LONG, BUT IF WE DON'T INCREASE OUR EXERCISE, WE WILL MAKE THIS GOOD NUTRITION LESS EFFECTIVE.

Let's also look a little closer at our children and how most, if not all gyms, don't welcome children to participate because what they have to offer is too intense for children to participate in on a regular basis. You will see even in a lot of the youth sports programs that those who participate in these sports and do weight lifting end up doing more damage to their body, as they are still growing. This can harm the growth plates and spine, therefore inhibiting the proper development and maturation of young to adolescent-age children. This can also lead to postural complications and developmental disturbances that will affect them for the rest of their life. The liability in gyms for children is much higher, which makes gyms want to impose these restrictions on children coming in, telling you that your children would not want to be a part of this. So, what do you do with your children to improve their exercise while still getting your own exercise increased as well? You do it with them right from your own home! It eliminates all the extra headache and fees of memberships and leaves enough time to get it all in the schedule.

So, the question we return to again—how can we improve a child's exercise and enhance their overall wellness? We can talk about nutrition all day long, but if we don't increase our exercise, we will make this good nutrition less effective. We must get our kids moving daily, as letting them sleep or lay around all day does them a huge disservice and depletes their body's natural ability to fight sickness because their immune system is decreased. As was already mentioned, this also reduces the function of their digestive system to properly digest the food that is eaten and produce the vital functions to pull out the vitamins and minerals and get proper blood flow throughout the body. But some parents don't know what to do to get their children moving, so let's make it simple.

"TO ENJOY THE GLOW OF GOOD HEALTH, YOU MUST EXERCISE."

GENE TUNNEY

First, encourage them to go outside and play more often. You don't see kids playing outside like you used to. They need to go out and be adventurous, build, climb, explore, and play hard to help increase their heart rate for a longer period of time. Moving the fingers and thumb on a controller does not have the same effect as physically getting out and doing something. Playing a good game of ball can also be something that can help them, or running laps and challenging them to do so. Why can't you join them in doing this to increase your heart rate as well, along with giving yourself the ability to get some extra vitamin D from the sun?

Okay, I get it—it's raining and gloomy out, or you have been gone all day and the kids can't go out and play. Fine, then what about doing something in the house, such as jump-roping, push-ups, jumping jacks, and many other things that could be done very easily indoors? In fact, this could be done while you are waiting for supper to cook in the oven. So many options can be considered, and so many more could be created in ways that could improve our overall workout just at home.

The excuses can pile up that we don't have time, or the kids aren't motivated to do it, or that it's like pulling a tooth to get them involved and energized to move more often. It may take a little more incentive to make it happen, because by human nature we aren't naturally eager to jump up and start doing a thousand pushups each day. But proper preparation and example can go a long way with our children, and we need to consider this as we begin to plan our day. Start off leading by example and encourage them to follow. If you aren't successful, create a home challenge where you challenge everyone in the house to see who can do the most in a month's time with a reward to follow. Soon it becomes a habit, not a challenge, and they will want to do it. In fact, you might even get the dog to try doing it, or even better, your spouse won't want to miss out on this challenge.

Once again, this doesn't have to be complex. As we implemented this into our routine it was always a small reward, and you can pick multiple activities that could be included in this challenge. It can be as basic as a pull up or running up and back down a flight of stairs. Anything is possible to create in your own home, even if you live in an apartment or in close proximity to your neighbors. This can even be done in a hotel! There really is no excuse for not doing something to improve the heart rate of yourself and your children, no matter where you are or what you are doing. There is no doubt that it does take time and dedication to make sure it will happen, but no excuse should outrule your approach to helping your health and improving the health of your children.

Many times, we build a little stubbornness when it comes to having to do something that we really don't want to do, and this is no different for our children. Sometimes they will find every way to get out of increasing their exercise, especially if their friends aren't doing it. This is where we have to be a little more clever and find ways we can do this without them really knowing. What respective task could you have them do around the house that would involve increasing their heart rate and getting them to move a little more? You sometimes have to think outside the box and be really creative in how you help them. It may even come into play that you pull in their friends and get them involved as well. Exercise won't hurt anyone, and the more you can do the better it will serve your family and the community as a whole. We think we have to keep this as a family project, but if you could help one child or another family, why not try to encourage them as well? It can turn into a natural community program. You never know what you could come up with if you don't step forward and try to help your family be a part of this and improve their overall activity.

The requirements are what get most people burned out, and you can read book after book to explain how long you should exercise and what you should do to make it the most effective. The key to the first step is to get moving and begin reducing your sedentary lifestyle and the lounging lifestyle of your kids. This starts by simply moving, and I will tell anyone that you cannot go from sitting still to a marathon runner overnight. You must build up to it. I know this may seem simple to most people, but it happens over and over that people want to get healthy, so they hit their exercise program running and burn out in a short amount of time. Why not take baby steps? Just as no baby starts running straight from the womb, why do you think you can do this with your exercise program?

You must start out slow with any program and work yourself up to where you want to be. This can easily be done with a starting plan of five minutes at a time. Maybe even push yourself and do

2-3 five-minute sessions throughout the day. Continue to do this for a week or so, with the plan to increase slowly. If you start with five minutes, then you can add additional five-minute increments to the routine you already have established. If you do multiple five-minute sessions, consider combining them into one or two workouts in a day's time before you start to add time. We have to picture changes in time at a slower rate when it comes to children. If you were to take them out on a twenty-minute jog right away, it would be hard to get them to come out again and do it all over the next day. This goes for everything we do to make a lifestyle change. Little by little, we will alter our life to adapt and make good choices to improve our health for the better.

We don't want to stay stagnant or do only five-minute workouts the rest of our life, but we all need a little challenge to be able to move to the next level. We have to grow, and whether we are talking about personal growth or exercise and healthy growth, we all need to improve. So, I challenge you to improve the health and wellness of your family as a whole, and the one aspect you are currently working on is to increase their movement each day. So, build on the five-minute rule and add ten minutes each day for the next week or two. Don't ever get content at this level, but continue to grow and add minutes every couple of weeks. When you hit the point of 20-30 minutes each day, then you can maintain and feel good about it. Now your body will adapt and become used to this routine.

You will want to change things from time to time or throughout the week, but maintaining at a daily exercise regime of 20-30 minutes will greatly improve your overall wellness. It will help you boost your immune system and the immune system of your children, and soon you will be able to look back and see that they may be performing better in school and they have totally new energy that is channeled in a new direction. This will not happen overnight, but will eventually be noticed over time and be impressive when you look back. Many exercise programs and exercise gurus tell you that you need to exercise only three times a week. While this is better than nothing, I strongly recommend that you take it to six days a week with one day of rest. You will find that so many will push their three days of exercise off, and soon they have to accomplish three days all in one. This can't and won't happen, leaving them skipping their exercise and soon forgetting it all together. Make it simple and work on it every single day, giving yourself and your family one designated day of rest each week. How much simpler can it get than that? We all could use a little more simplicity in our lives.

You can look at this as a challenge to create your own unique exercise program that works for you and your family. There can always be excuses made, such as saying that you don't have exercise equipment like a treadmill or stationary bike, or that there isn't a place to do exercise in your own home, that you have to build something and you know it won't happen. This is where you are letting the excuses of life get the best of you, and you prefer letting your health go over improving it for yourself and your family. You must be creative and become your own personal trainer. We all would like to have the advantage of having someone coach us each and every step of the way, but we have to take some initiative to begin and actually do something.

Exercise is where you can begin this creativity and build your own program. Really, you don't need anything to create an outstanding workout in your home. You can do push-ups, sit ups, jumping jacks, lunges, curls, jump rope, running in place, stairs, and the list goes on and on. You can even add hiking, swimming, biking, and jogging to your routine to change it up so you aren't doing the same thing all the time. If you are wanting to go someplace with the family, consider walking or biking there instead of driving. You can run in place as if you were jogging and get your children to run right next to you at the same time. Dribble a ball around on a hard floor as if you are playing basketball, but keep moving. See how easy this can be? You can even do squats as you pick up the house, and whoever picks up the most stuff wins the challenge. Even while you are cooking, you can easily throw in a little exercise for both parents and children. While you wait to brown your meat, you can put a can of something on the ground and pick it up and put it back, repeating over and over and making a little game of it. It's not a 100 lb. weight, but you are in motion, improving your circulation and respiration to improve your health. Focus on that, and soon you will see your fatigue slowly disappear and your energy will be higher than it's ever been before.

"THOSE WHO THINK THEY HAVE NOT TIME FOR BODILY EXERCISE WILL SOONER OR LATER HAVE TO FIND TIME FOR ILLNESS."

EDWARD STANLEY

The whole message to take away from this is to not make your exercise program too complex. Instead, just simplify it so you are in motion and do something you can accomplish each day. Set yourself up to get moving and include the whole family so everyone can get moving as well to improve so many of the bodily functions on a daily basis. We all need to improve on how we increase our heart rate and improve our deep breathing, clearing out the toxic air and oxygenating our blood more, which then brings more oxygen to our brain and the rest of the organs in our body. What if toxins have built up in our body and we cannot process and filter our blood, leaving us with other complications that we don't even know we have? We will talk about this in another chapter about toxins, but if we bring in more pure oxygen and focus on improving all the areas of our body, we will better remove some of these toxins and help our overall function of life. Our stress levels will decrease, and we can handle day-to-day tasks with more ease than before.

You might not believe this will make a difference, but take the challenge by giving it a try. It will be exciting to look back in a few weeks to see your progress and how the performance of your children in school and overall behavior changes daily. See how your mood and perspective on life changes and how you handle the stress that you are presented with. These all can happen with a little movement and making these changes in our life with a little exercise.

"Drinking water is like washing out your insides.
The water will cleanse the system, fill you up, decrease your
caloric load and improve the function of all your tissues."

– Kevin Stone

9

WATER

"Are you drinking enough?"

THIS TOPIC SEEMS so basic that it gets overlooked most of the time. Very few people seem to talk about it, even though it has such a large contributing factor to our natural good health. We don't drink enough water in our life to meet the demands of our body. Tiredness is one of the most common symptoms of dehydration, and how often in a day do we feel tired or draggy? If you ask anyone, they will probably tell you over and over that they drink a lot of water or they aren't thirsty, so they don't worry about not getting enough. But do we consider that this may really be a cause of not enough water? This comes into play when we talk about the health and wellness of the family, especially our children. When our children ask for a drink, what do we give them—water, or some other liquid like milk, pop, or juice? They don't drink enough water at meals or throughout the day. If we are feeling tired in the middle of the day, do we reach for a cup of coffee or a sugary drink?

This isn't enough to meet our body's demands, and without really knowing we are damaging our organs and body, and it will reflect on our ongoing performance long term.

There are numerous benefits of drinking plenty of water. It can eliminate fatigue, help you focus more sharply, support healthy skin, and cleanse the kidneys. How do you think we rehydrate the cells in our body? By drinking water, of course! It also balances body fluids and supports healthy digestion and elimination. Have you ever wondered why your children are constipated? Have you ever thought about how little water they are getting? Sure, they may drink a lot during the day, but how much of what they drink is pure water? Ideally our whole family should be drinking a minimum of half the body's weight in ounces each day. So, if a child weighs forty pounds they should be drinking approximately twenty ounces of water each day.

> THERE ARE NUMEROUS BENEFITS OF DRINKING PLENTY OF WATER. IT CAN ELIMINATE FATIGUE, HELP YOU FOCUS MORE SHARPLY, SUPPORT HEALTHY SKIN, AND CLEANSE THE KIDNEYS. HOW DO YOU THINK WE REHYDRATE THE CELLS IN OUR BODY? BY DRINKING WATER, OF COURSE!

We have to make these changes and work daily to build up our water intake so that we can run and function properly. Depending on the resource you look at, it is noted that our body contains about 80-85% water. If we run this dry, how do we expect to work properly and function like our body really should? This is something that once again does not change overnight, nor should it, but we can build this up over time and soon we can properly run smoother like we need to. Just think—if you don't give your car the right amount of oil, soon it will stop running. Our body is no different, so we simply have to keep the tank full of water so we can physically run and function. If we don't, it won't take long and we will start having more and more issues that will slow us down.

Pure water is one of the most natural and well-supplied nutrients that we can give our body plenty of on a daily basis. Not all water is the same or the best for us, as some contains higher level of toxicities. Overall, most areas have a good source or two of purified water that we can enjoy. We must consume enough water that we can support our bodies. How do we do this as parents and then make sure that we get enough in our children? Having a set glass or cup so you know the amount you are drinking is always helpful. So many will say that they are drinking a lot, but when they start to keep a record of it, they realize they are drinking less than they thought they were. I would surmise that this is happening to most people, and we need to find a good container of some sort and consistently drink from that bottle or glass. Even keeping track can be helpful so you know how many ounces you have in that cup; it can help you keep a better record. In order to help keep track of what your kids are drinking, let them pick out a fun-looking water bottle, determine how many ounces that holds, and have your child put tick marks or designate in a certain area how many of those bottles they drank that day. Obviously if they are older, they may not want to participate in this method, and you may need to come up with another way they feel comfortable with. The key isn't to babysit them on their water-drinking abilities, but more importantly to help hold each other accountable to drinking the designated amount of water.

There is something that you need to take note of, and that is to not drink all the required water in one sitting or on the first day you start upping your water intake. This will cause you to spend your day in the bathroom, leaving you very discouraged or wondering what is wrong with you. It takes a gradual buildup of drinking more until your body can support the full amount that it really demands. It does take time for your body to regulate as it is, but doing this all at once will destroy your hopes of making this a lifestyle change. This is most critical for our children as we help them begin to increase their tolerance and build up that fluid level in their body. This is one level that many families struggle with, as their children are far from having even close to the right amount of water intake each time, and are supplementing with sugar-filled beverages such as soda, energy drinks, juice, or milk. We have to eliminate these from our children's choice selection and reserve them for very special times. We cannot be unrealistic and think that we can remove everything from their diet and not give them anything to enjoy as a treat once in a great while. It doesn't work to yank all other drinks away and expect our family to only drink water for the rest of their life. In another chapter we will discuss this so we can really understand the point that we have to have a plan to follow in order to make our children successful and keep our family striving for the best. Water is part of this, and we have to step them down from other beverages and fill them up with the proper fluids that they need.

We can optimize this plan for our family by having organized water bottles sitting around ready for each day so we can begin this journey and follow through with it. If our children have to depend on finding their own bottle or source of water, they are less likely to fulfill the required amount of water each day. Our bodies run on water and we use it to biochemically function and metabolize our foods, transport waste out of our system, and move blood around the body. Not to mention, we cushion our joints and supply nutrient support to our muscles. As was mentioned, when around 80% (this number is different in every resource you look at) of our body is water, we need to furnish it with what it needs. When we sweat, that is wicking out of the body and not going back in. When we urinate, that is expelling liquid out but not back in. If you want to maintain the most adequate amount of good water in our body, you must re-fill the tank each day. This does not mean a glass each day; this means you get the adequate amount each day on top of your glass at meals. This does not have to be complex. Simply have a water bottle ready and filled, with the number of bottles they need written on the bottom of each one. Then they have access to an easy way to fill and use over and over again so that there is no excuse for their water intake.

"WATER IS THE MOST NEGLECTED NUTRIENT IN YOUR DIET, BUT ONE OF THE MOST VITAL."
JULIA CHILD

There are times that we don't enjoy drinking water, and this can be hard because so many turn to other beverages, such as soda or coffee. This gives you liquid but also acts against the body, causing you to become more and more dehydrated to the point that you need to be drinking more fluids on top of the caffeine you are drinking. If you want to say you are drinking caffeine-free soda, great for you. But the sugars in this diet soda will affect you worse than the caffeine, which now makes it ineffective. Drinking juice, unless it is 100% natural, will also provide sugars that will drive up inflammation as was mentioned in the sugar section of this book.

We have to decide, are we going to go all the way and give our body what it needs, or go halfway and only do part of it, not utilizing it to the fullest? If you have to have that coffee or soda and your kids pick up that habit with you, then do your body a favor and drink an additional eight ounces of water for every cup or can you drink of anything else. This needs to be the rule, or your water intake will fall short every time and won't allow you to function at a high quality as you should. We have to nourish our bodies with good nutrients that can properly be carried throughout our body, with water being that source. We have such great elements that our body can use. Why not keep all those contaminations out and flush our body daily with a pure substance that can be utilized without being a detriment to the body?

"THE BEST SIX DOCTORS: SUNSHINE, WATER, REST, AIR, EXERCISE & DIET."
UNKNOWN

So many complain that they cannot stand water and what it tastes like, and this can be a huge factor that is slowing the consumption of water. Water is designed to be odorless and tasteless, and if we do not have these two attributes, then we do not have pure water. This happens in our town and it taste like chlorine. It makes one wonder how helpful this really could be for the body and what other toxins are in it that could hinder our body. This should not be considered drinkable water, and we need to find a good source of pure water to drink. If this is not possible, then add good nutrients such as lemons, limes, strawberries, mint leaves, cucumbers, or anything else that could add natural flavor to enhance your drinking experience. It can be really fun for kids to see the variety of color in their bottles and it makes them more enthusiastic to drink it. Also, a good source of pure essential oils can be helpful to drop in one or two drops to add flavor. This makes it better to drink and helps purify the body with good sources of lemons and limes. Mint leaves from the garden can also be steeped and drank as an iced tea to get more water consumption in. This does have some caffeine, but does help get better water consumption in the body. Try some of these alternative ways to always increase your water consumption and continue to always consume more and more water.

To make this as basic as we can, let's review what needs to be done when it comes to water and drinking enough. We should have a designated water supply that is good for the whole family to drink. This should be as free from toxins as possible and be enjoyable for all to drink. Then have your specific drinking containers that show how much each person should drink. This is configured by taking your weight and dividing it in half, using that number as the ounces per day that you should drink. If you aren't close to that number, then keep building up each day, not doing it all in one setting. If water isn't palatable for you to drink, add any flavor of fruit or vegetable to make it more desirable, also keeping essential oils in mind as a great source as well. Then maintain this level daily and you will see how it can improve your brain function, energy, and daily bodily functions. We need water to make our engine go, through the blood vascular system, lymphatic system, and muscles/joints. When it consumes 80% of your body, it is a bit important.

Really take an inventory of how much water you and your children are drinking on a daily basis. We tend to get too busy to recognize how much we are really taking in, or if our kids are really drinking enough. We have to have a way to get the good nutrients into our cells and the bad toxins out of our body. We know that if we do not keep a car's engine cool through our coolant, it will become overheated and ruin the engine. This is the same for our bodies as well and we have to do all we can. We sweat to keep our bodies cool and to remove toxins out of our body. We urinate, which then flushes the liver and kidneys, removing all the poor toxins out of the body as well, purifying our bodies. We need this fluid in our brain, as it helps cushion and provides the environment that our body needs for the brain and the spinal cord. It helps to supply fluid to the joints, just as oil does to a working engine to make the parts move better.

All in all, we must have this vital component in our body and well-supplied so we all run well. Our kids are not getting the water supply they need to do this, driving the risk of their digestive systems not functioning right and their brains to become foggy and forgetful. They play hard and we may work hard, making the body work as it should, but we have to refill the tank so it can be utilized for the next day. Running on empty can only go so far before we start ruining the body and having bigger issues to deal with. Please make sure your family is getting plenty of water each day!

All those toxins in your body are blocking the healing process: amalgams in your teeth, an infection, a yeast overgrowth, fluoride, environmental toxins, pesticides, herbicides, and heavy metals. They are a roadblock to your healing."

– Dr. Danial Nuzum, D.O., NMD

10

TOXINS

What is killing us?

THIS ONE WORD SEEMS to be something that is very dangerous. When we see it on a household cleaner, we are extremely cautious while using it. But when we add this label to something that your child may have in them, we don't seem to be as concerned with it and dismiss it on a daily basis. Toxins are everywhere and make it near impossible to escape the dangers that surround us all the time, especially when we realize that most of the toxins we have in our body come from the food we eat. When you go to the grocery store, do you know exactly where all the fresh vegetables come from and how they were treated before they arrive into your community? Think about the crops that surround us and produce much of the food we eat, or what the animals we consume eat as they are raised. Most of these crops are treated, often with very dangerous herbicides and pesticides.

An example is the glyphosate (that's in the herbicide roundup) that the corn both we and animals eat is treated with. It is very harmful to our digestive system and causes an alarming number of issues. We harvest crops which grow in soil that has been treated for years, creating a toxic buildup over time. We then receive these grains and consume them, not thinking anything about it. The same goes for the animals that are raised for meat and who consume the grains and even the pasture. This has been treated as well, and they ingest the toxins found on these plants, taking them into the body. Our wonderful body digests this food and removes the dangerous toxins, which we hope to get expelled out of our body and into the waste.

That isn't the case all the time, as often our gastrointestinal tract is compromised and we absorb more toxins into our bloodstream than we thought or even know. Thankfully, it is then filtered out in the liver. So, we may think these toxins are either filtered out in the waste or through our liver and get pulled out some way, we never have to worry about it. Then why is it such a big deal? Even though the liver can filter out these toxins, they start to accumulate in the liver, building up a toxic environment over time and spilling over into other areas of the body. These are heavy metal toxicities that cannot pass out of our body at this point. We cannot process them, leaving them in an area that is less functional and causing damage to the liver, essentially being passed to other areas of the body such as the highly vascularized brain. This then can alter the function of our brain, and high enough levels can decrease our brain function, causing our long- and short-term memory to fail. It can alter our behavior and moods daily, and we end up blaming it on stress or hormones. Our children can also suffer from it, and it could cause them to feel unwell without really knowing what the issue might be, but more importantly, you may recognize alteration in their behavior and performance in school. This so often gets diagnosed as a neurological/behavioral issue, and they get put on medication to control it or have to be pulled out of school. This isn't their fault, as there are no other approaches or solutions offered to these families.

Consider the fact that if these toxins are built up in the body, they also affect the brain, and they mainly consist of heavy metals like arsenic, lead, mercury, and several others. What impact could these have on your child's brain? Heavy metals will slow down the brain's function and poison the blood, inhibiting the oxygen-rich blood's capacity to reproduce the red blood cells effectively and leaving the highly functioning brain depleted and starving for more, then killing off some of the neurological pathways that we use every single day to function, especially mood and behavior.

> **"BY CLEANSING YOUR BODY ON A REGULAR BASIS AND ELIMINATING AS MANY TOXINS AS POSSIBLE FROM YOUR ENVIRONMENT, YOUR BODY CAN BEGIN TO HEAL ITSELF, PREVENT DISEASE, AND BECOME STRONGER AND MORE RESILIENT THAN YOU EVER DREAMED POSSIBLE!"**
>
> DR. EDWARD GROUP

These toxins/heavy metals can and will affect each person and child differently, so don't be alarmed or worry about whether this may or may not be the issue. We have to recognize that this could be a potential issue and understand what steps we as a family can take. Remember, we have to build a strong immunity in ourselves and our families in order to fight off the common bugs or sicknesses that they will get. Don't walk around with a mask on all the time, thinking that after every breath or step your child may take, you need to wash them off–likewise with the food they put in their mouth. We have to recognize that if they are suffering from conditions we cannot figure out, we need to look a little deeper into what might be causing it and understand that they may need these toxins cleansed from the body.

"TODAY, MORE THAN 95% OF CHRONIC DISEASE IS CAUSED BY FOOD CHOICE, TOXIC FOOD INGREDIENTS, NUTRITIONAL DEFICIENCIES, AND LACK OF PHYSICAL EXERCISE."

MIKE ADAMS

Traveling back a little into where we can pick up some of these toxins, I want to discuss that they are everywhere. From the paint we use, to the glue in the carpet that is laid in our houses, to the bug sprays we use, to the plastic cups we drink out of, to the treatment of the water we drink. Everything has the potential to have toxins in it, and we can worry ourselves sick that our children will develop a nasty cancer and die in six months. That is not the case, and we don't have to be alarmed every second of our lives. Instead simply consider what you are using and where it might be coming from. Could you get better-grown produce out of your own garden that your children could eat, or buy meat sources that have been grass-fed and the farmer knows that nothing has been sprayed on the fields in which they were harvested? Let's face it—we all can't have our own garden in our back yard, as some may live in a high-rise and/or they cannot afford the high-end organic foods at the market. Don't lose perspective in thinking all is lost and your child is going to die and you caused it. Think outside the box a little and determine how you can grow or purchase good healthy foods at a lower cost for your children.

There are so many ways you can grow fresh greens right in your tiny porch or patio, or even great sprouts in the corner of your kitchen where you know what has been exposed to them. However, let's make this even more simplified and know that when you purchase good foods from the markets, you can wash them in vinegar water for a short amount of time and rinse off a lot of these toxins, removing them and making these foods much healthier for your children and family to consume.

Stressing about every item that your family may come into contact with will only drive an increased amount of stress in your life and deplete your ability to function properly. Then the resources will have to be applied to you, and this all becomes ineffective all the way around. Let your children play in the dirt and walk barefoot outside. Let them explore in areas that are safe, but maybe aren't areas that we feel have always been clean and safe from germs. This will help build up a stronger immunity and prepare them to face a flu or cold season so much better. Just remember, if you or any one in your family feel that they aren't acting in a manner that is normal or you feel that your children continue to feel sick or act out, consider looking into their heavy metal toxicity and removing any that may be hindering their function. This can be easily done by sending a hair sample in for analysis to see what may be contained in the hair. After all, the skin tries to wick out any toxins in the body, and so if we provide a sampling closer to the surface we can determine what toxins may be trying to find their way out of the body. If you have a higher level at the surface, it is most certain that you will have a higher level in your liver that is trying to get expelled but cannot.

In the event that you feel you need to cleanse out these toxins(I recommend doing so as a family once or twice a year, just to clean them out so they do not build up), I would consult a qualified individual that has experience in this and can make the right recommendations to you based off of what your exposure and/or conditions might be. This can be simply done by cleaning up your diet and removing the processed foods, healing the gastrointestinal tract, and flushing out the liver, kidneys, and bladder with increased amount of water. There may be a cleanse protocol that may be used in order to better assist pulling out those heavier toxins that normally may not be able to be expelled without the extra help from the body. Again, consult a professional before you try to tackle something like this and help reduce the risk of further harm to the body by not having the right combination to remove these toxins.

Toxins are everywhere and in everything, from the sources of food that we eat to the products that we use on a daily basis. Try to reduce your exposure by washing your food products properly and with vinegar and letting them dry before you consume them. Also consider switching the health and household products that you have around the house to ones that are more natural, or even learning how to make your own so you know what you are putting into the clean or health products you are taking. Spend more time outside getting fresh air, and reduce the time you spend in cramped, enclosed indoor spaces, allowing the body to process and remove as many toxins as you can by flushing with plenty of water and exercise.

One can do everything they can possibly think of and try to live cautiously, but we cannot survive in a bubble. Our bodies are wonderfully made by our Creator, and He knew what He was doing when we were created. He allowed the body to cleanse out many of the toxins through our skin and urinary system, but we have to provide the environment for this to happen. So before you get all consumed in how you are going to do the next detox, consider providing your body and your children with the proper tools to increase water so they can sweat. Then encourage increased exercise so they can sweat this out, cleansing out these toxins. If this is done along with improving your gastrointestinal tract lining, then you don't have anything to worry about. This can be done first by removing the irritants that we are consuming with processed foods and sugars, and replacing them with higher levels of

TOXINS ARE EVERYWHERE AND IN EVERYTHING, FROM THE SOURCES OF FOOD THAT WE EAT TO THE PRODUCTS THAT WE USE ON A DAILY BASIS.

good vegetables and some fruit. A good probiotic, which will introduce the good bacteria into the gastrointestinal tract, will help process our foods and produce an environment that is healthy and ready to digest and pull the good nutrients from the foods we consume. Also, diffusing purifying essential oils and using proper cleansing essential oils can help clean out the air in our homes from extra toxins that otherwise we would be breathing in on a daily basis. Stressing over the toxin content can be the worst thing you could do as a parent, but acknowledging it and trying to do what you can to clean up will go a long way toward reducing the buildup that may come over time. Remember that building up toxin levels to a capacity we cannot handle doesn't happen overnight, but it is a gradual increase over time, and will start to affect us and our children.

*"One of the biggest tragedies of human civilization
is the precedents of chemical therapy over nutrition."*

- Dr. Royal Lee

11

SUPPLEMENTS/OILS/HERBS/TINCTURES
Treat the body from the outside in or the inside out.

THIS TOPIC IS VERY controversial depending on what you have heard or personally experienced. If you are from the allopathic medicine community, you may not be able to relate to this, as prescription medication is the only way to heal in that community. Now, I must preface this by saying we need each other to make the body function as a whole. And I want to express that there are times when alternative ways through supplementation of herbs are not always the way to go. Trauma would be an example of this, as when someone is severely hurt with a gaping wound or has broken bones, there are no number of supplements or herbs that can patch up or set bones properly. As much as we may not want to go to the emergency department, this is a must and we are very thankful for the wonderful training and care that can be received in such cases. We have to know the limits for our family and respect each medical establishment for what they have to offer for each specific case.

We can do all we can to try to help our families and children for common illnesses and overall health, but you have to know when it is out of your control and depend on the professionals to do what they are trained in.

We have to understand that these alternative forms of healing the body are exactly what they are stated as. We should use them as "supplements" to what we eat, which gives another prime example of why what we eat and what we put in our mouths is very important. If we put the right foods into our mouths, eliminating those foods that can cause more damage, we should be able to maintain a healthy way of living without a multitude of supplements or herbs to treat our bodies. A very common mistake is for mothers to read how a certain supplement or vitamin is supposed to help one ailment, and then another supplement helps a different issue that is present in the family. Pretty soon, the whole family is taking so many supplements, tinctures, and oils that do more damage than good for them. We should not be overdosing ourselves with all these supplements especially when we don't take the time to heal our gastrointestinal tract and have proper absorption. What so many people don't realize is that if they are taking so many extra things, their body cannot absorb all of this. If we don't get to the root cause of the issue and heal the gut microbiome first by eating properly, supplementation will be pointless as the valuable nutrients won't be absorbed into the body but will be passed through without doing anything. This happens over and over for many who take a whole list of these beneficial nutrients but won't take the time to eat properly and devote to truly healing the body with proper nutrition.

If we are really eating properly, we should need very little extra supplementation for our families. Something we need to understand is that even with whole, organic foods, we still won't have the quality or amount of nutrients that we would have gotten from the same foods years ago. That said, some supplementation may be necessary, but we need to be very picky on what we are putting into our mouths as far as supplements and what brand we are using. Sure, there are thousands of different brands out in the world today, and we have to recognize that not all brands and types of supplements are the same. Just because you found some cheap vitamin C doesn't mean that it is healthy and good for us to consume on a regular basis.

The big news that so many people do not know is the fact that supplement companies, oils, herbs, and tinctures are not regulated by the Food and Drug Administration (FDA). This organization is used to mandate many of the foods that we consume, making sure they are human-approved and provide an adequate support for the body. Now this organization also regulates pharmaceutical companies and drugs, and we feel safer because of it. Unfortunately, without getting into a long political discussion, money can grant winning certification to about anything in the pharmaceutical drugs industry, even with the many horrible side effects. The alternative route is not always regulated by the FDA, which can be a very good thing, but also can make it tricky to understand all that goes into them. With this said, not all supplements, oils, and tinctures are created equal and should be treated this way. Please be very picky when it comes to these items, and don't assume a frugal mindset is the way to go by making it cheap for your family. Buy quality and know what you are getting before you start taking them, or they will be no different than the damaging foods that you are putting into your family's body.

The first thing to look for in a supplement is to make sure that it is a whole food-based supplement. This is best because you will know that it is real food that is being taken. Taking a step further to get organic whole food-based supplements is optimal, but not always realistic for everyone. What you don't want to do is grab something that is cheap and seems to be the same thing as all the other supplements, when you have no idea what's inside it. Just like processed foods, there can be a lot of fillers inside supplements that give you a very small portion of the real thing and the remainder is filled with synthetic materials that cannot be processed in your body, and in fact damage your body more.

Would you sit down and chew on some plastic and expect it to be digested and processed through your body, providing excellent nutritional value? Of course not! So why would you put supplements containing synthetics into your body as good nutritional supplementation? An example of a calcium supplement you would want to stay away from would be one that has calcium carbonate in it. This is one of the cheapest forms of calcium, derived from eggshells, rocks, pearls, shells, etc. Calcium carbonate requires extra stomach acid to be absorbed, as it isn't highly bioavailable. Research warns that excessive consumption could cause poor digestion and be hazardous. As another example, consider the synthetic form of vitamin B1, thiamine mononitrate. This vitamin is not easily absorbed either because it is fat soluble, making it more difficult for the body to remove. Natural thiamine is non-toxic, but synthetic versions are and could cause allergic reactions, kidney problems, or even infertility. Do these vitamins sound like what you want to be giving to your family on a daily basis? Take the time to do your own research so you can read and understand what the labels are.

We don't need to complicate this anymore, other than to realize that filler synthetics found in our supplements are exactly what they sound like, and they are very cheap to put in. That makes the product so affordable and draws so many more to buy it. Makes sense, right?! However, we can't digest these synthetics. They damage our body systems, introducing more toxins into the body. So when you take such a small amount of a good product such as vitamin C and you fill the rest with extra fillers, you would have to take a lot more of that vitamin C to actually get what you need. But you are also filling your body with extra toxins coming from the synthetics. These synthetic vitamins are like fake vitamins and actually can be doing more harm than good. Be properly informed and don't waste your money on products that really won't help you in the end. That's why so many people may start taking supplements but eventually give up, saying that they do not notice a difference whether they take them or not.

We have looked into the production a little more and understand the marketing tactics of any product. The problem with pharmaceutical drugs is the point that nobody challenges what might be inside and they take them because they are "FDA-approved." Have you ever read the list of possible side effects that are handed out with each prescription? These are killing our generation today. We take a drug, have a side effect, then take another drug to treat that issue, and the cycle repeats itself over and over. The same can be said with synthetic supplements, and you continue to take them for life without knowing that they could be harming you long term.

We often get two responses out of this when people are informed saying, "Well, I'm not going to take these any longer and I'm just going to eat well." The other side looks into the research, understanding what their body needs and knows what they need to take. Now, it makes sense why some would say that they are no longer going to take supplements when they don't feel a difference; they are probably not getting enough of a good thing to make a difference in their body. So they stop, but they don't change their diet habits either and their health starts to decline.

We supplement in order to have the nutrients that our body needs on a daily basis. Because of the many modifications that happen in our food supply today in order to make bigger and better foods, we have lost a lot of the many valuable nutrients we once had. So now more than ever you have to consume higher levels of vitamin C, vitamin D, zinc, and other highly valuable supplements on a daily basis. Just because you have a supplement doesn't allow for the excuse that you don't have to eat as much spinach. It doesn't work that way; no matter how many supplements you take, you pull more nutrients out of the foods that you eat than taking it in pill form. We have to use supplements as they are intended—as a supplement to our diet. Add additional nutrients to foods that we used to get, but no longer get because of the modifications. There really isn't anything we can do to enhance the quality of food we are eating because it has been genetically modified over time, and we cannot get that back. Sure, we should try

> **WE SUPPLEMENT IN ORDER TO HAVE THE NUTRIENTS THAT OUR BODY NEEDS ON A DAILY BASIS. BECAUSE OF THE MANY MODIFICATIONS THAT HAPPEN IN OUR FOOD SUPPLY TODAY TO MAKE BIGGER AND BETTER FOODS, WE HAVE LOST A LOT OF THE MANY VALUABLE NUTRIENTS WE ONCE HAD.**

to grow our own vegetables if we can. If not, consume those that go back to organic basis to try to get the highest nutrient content that we can. But supplementation is still necessary to make sure we have the proper levels of vitamins and nutrients that the body needs to function properly.

Now, we know we need to supplement, but how do I know I'm getting the highest level of nutrients that I can when I take supplements? This is a great question, and it's a simple one to answer. Go back to the basics and find whole food, nutrient-dense supplements. They are more expensive because they have to be grown, harvested, and processed down to powder form or whatever form they need to be. With synthetics, we can dump it right into the factory and that's it. There is no growing process or much time to create it, so it definitely is cheaper, and we have to understand that.

Whole food supplements are exactly what they sound like. They contain whole foods that are ground up and many times dehydrated or processed to make it into a suitable form so we can capsulate or tablet them. Some nutrients from this process will always be lost. But in the end, it is much more condensed, giving us the equivalent of what we would receive by eating 2-3 times the amount in food (which would be nearly impossible). Also, many of the companies that create these whole food supplements grow their own foods and process them themselves. They know what is going into them and they produce only the highest quality. If you have had the opportunity to travel to a supplement facility and see this process from farm to tablet/capsule, it can be very rewarding to know how it is done.

One thing that needs to be mentioned when looking at whole food supplements, you also need to be aware of is the label. Look at the label, and it won't be the same label that you see on traditional supplements. Why? Because whole food supplements will have a food label on them since that is exactly what they are and that's why they need a food label over a supplement label. That can be one quick thing to notice when you are shopping for supplements. First, is it more expensive. Second, if it says whole food on the label. And third, if it has a food label on the side. If you are unsure of what that looks like, look on the side of your bag of carrots next time and you will see the difference. Not to mention, you can actually recognize all the ingredients found inside of the supplement and know that it would be nutrient rich for you to take them.

Think about it for a minute: Wouldn't you rather put a supplement in your body that has the same label as your package of spinach or radishes? That is how we need to look at this because when you take cheap supplements from any store, you are essentially tossing money out. Most of the time these poor supplements are ending up in your sewer system and providing more damage to your body.

We've now discussed that we need to spend more time checking out our supplements and making sure they are whole food supplements, filled with real nutrients for ourselves and the family. That's not hard to do, but is something that you need to consider. Now, what should we be taking and giving our children so they are getting everything that they need? That is the biggest question, and it is impossible to give a conclusive list. Often it depends on who you talk with and what they recommend, which drives you to try multiple things and often become discouraged as a parent because the list becomes extensive. Consider starting with the basics and build from that. Give your children and the entire family a good source of a well-balanced whole food multivitamin to start off with. This is where one can start, as we can distribute the well-rounded good nutrients that are found in that multivitamin. One that is rich in whole food vegetables where they have taken the entire vegetable and ground it up, providing deep nutrients that are found in the skins or peels. The same can be considered with fruits as well, and often we don't get the deep variety that many of these supplements contain. We also peel or discard the outer layer that has so many rich nutrients that give us higher levels of the vitamins and minerals we can't pull from food. So many of these also can be catered to our children, and they can enjoy eating them on a daily basis, giving them so much more than we can offer in just food alone.

Now that we understand what we need to look for when searching for supplements, how do we know what supplements to take? We are constantly surrounded with the elements of our environment, and as much as we try to eat the very best that we can, we still wander into un-nutrient environments that can damage our gastrointestinal bacteria, which then damages our gastrointestinal lining, leaving us nutrient-depleted because we don't have the absorption that we need. So, a proper probiotic would be on the top of the list for supplements that we should consider having in the medicine cabinet. By taking a good probiotic, we can bring these bacteria back into our gut and help establish this perfect balance that helps us properly digest the good foods we take in. When searching for a great probiotic, look for one that has a good prebiotic and a probiotic combined. This will allow the prebiotic to condition the gastrointestinal tract to utilize the probiotic, making it much more effective. Don't take this wrong—a good probiotic will be beneficial, but having the prebiotic takes the effectiveness to the next level, and it only enhances the outcome in the end. Many of you might find that you have to find a good probiotic in the refrigerated section and that you must keep it in that environment, as it contains a live culture. This may be helpful and makes you feel that you are giving them a better product than one that is stored in your cupboard, and that might be so. However, so many forget to give their children this supplement when it is in a different location and/or allow it to become outdated. The shelf life of these live cultures is much shorter. Without you realizing it, you may end up giving yourself and family something that is ineffective or even damaging to the gastrointestinal lining. Consider taking one that is again whole foods that are set up in a way that it contains all the bacteria that you need, but does not have to be stored in the refrigerator. These can be just as effective in the long run, and you can place it right beside the others, helping you as a parent to be able to remember it much better. Let's face it, we all could use a little more simplicity in our lives.

OUR BRAIN NEEDS FAT TO FUNCTION PROPERLY, SO IF WE ARE LIVING ON A LOW-FAT DIET, WE ARE ACTUALLY STARVING OUR BRAINS BY DEPLETING THEM OF THE PROPER NUTRITION TO GROW AND DEVELOP.

For years it has been ingrained into society that we need a low-fat diet so we don't gain weight. Well, the opposite of this is actually true. Our brain needs fat to function properly, so if we are living on a low-fat diet, we are actually starving our brains by depleting them of the proper nutrition to grow and develop. It is important to supplement with essential omega-3 fatty acids which is best accomplished by taking a well-sourced fish oil. Most of us are not able to feast on high-quality, fresh, deep-sea fish daily in order get these higher levels of fats that we need in our body. It improves the neurological connections in our brain, making the right and left brain work more effectively with each other and improving the response time within our brain. It helps to reduce the cardiovascular risk of arthrosclerosis in the vessels, bringing down much of our cholesterol and triglycerides to a healthy level. Now, most families don't have to worry about this, as their children aren't struggling with their cholesterol or in danger of a heart attack or stroke. Remember though, these conditions are affecting those younger and younger all the time. So if we don't start now and pass this information onto our children, they may be affected, or your future grandchildren may be affected. Health is inherited and passed on from one generation to the next, and we have to do our part to instill in our children what is most important now so they can carry that healthy lifestyle on for the rest of their life.

HEALTH IS INHERITED AND PASSED ON FROM ONE GENERATION TO THE NEXT, AND WE HAVE TO DO OUR PART TO INSTILL IN OUR CHILDREN WHAT IS MOST IMPORTANT NOW SO THEY CAN CARRY THAT HEALTHY LIFESTYLE ON FOR THE REST OF THEIR LIFE.

Not all fish is created equal, so it is very important to make sure you choose a quality omega oil supplement. Let's face it, many families don't enjoy the levels of fish or even the omega-3 sources needed. So they need to be supported with supplementation in order to get the proper levels. Look for a good source that isn't the cheapest. After all, if you buy cheap fish from the market that has been farm-raised, most likely you are going to get fish that contain high levels of mercury, causing a toxic buildup in your body and leaving damage to your brain instead of helping it. Get a good solid fish oil that may say it is taken from deep sea sources, and not farm raised. Two sources that you can consider would be to take a tuna omega or cod liver oil. As a caution, some family members or children may have reactions to higher doses of fish omega oils. Please make sure that you use small doses for younger children, or use a good source of sesame seed oil or plant-based omega-3 oils instead, as there don't seem to be problems with these.

Starting with the basics, we talked about a good probiotic, omega-3 oil, and then to add one more would be a whole-food multivitamin. We can start out as simple as these three to add a supportive nutritional base to our wellness. After 90 days of eating well and taking proper supplements, you can then determine if you can see a difference in yourself and your family. Aside from the basic three supplements to start with, here are a few other ones that you may want to consider if it is determined that there is a deficiency. If you don't get outside or have children that don't get out in the sun, you can consider supplementing with a good vitamin D that would help improve their overall immune system and body functions. Many times, people in general don't get out and get enough sunlight that can provide a good dose of vitamin D. If there is a lack of vitamin D, sometimes supplementation may be necessary. Having the proper amount of vitamin D can enhance so much in our bodies, from our brain, to the gut, to healthy hair and nails. Calcium and magnesium could be other good vitamins that are commonly lacking in individuals today. Muscle cramps or soreness are common symptoms of the lack of calcium and magnesium. It is best to take these two vitamins simultaneously for better absorption in the body.

A few more that we can consider keeping on our shelf would be again a good source of vitamin C, or any good immune supportive supplements that one can take when they start to feel ill and hopefully boost the immune system. So often, we wait until we are feeling really ill with full-fledged symptoms before we start taking anything to combat the sickness, and by that point it is really too late to keep it at bay. For the best results, you need to take these early on as soon as you slightly start to feel something. It often helps to hand out the immune boosting supplements to everyone in your family that might come in contact with the individual that isn't feeling well. It isn't normally recommended to just give supplements to them, but if you can reduce the risk from a sickness passing through everyone in the family, what a huge benefit this would be. Concluding the list can be a host of many other supplements, which in the end can help and often are found to treat specific conditions or symptoms. These would be the basic supplements that would be encouraged for families to have in their cupboard.

We now have the supplements, and we are ready to help our family with their overall health. This is a great place to be at. One thing that comes up so often is, how much should you take? So many will refrain from taking anything because they don't know what to take or how much. There are also rumors that some have died from taking too much of a supplement, and that it builds up in the body, causing a child to become toxic. The occurrence of this is rare to none, especially if each one is following the dosage directions on the bottle or the manufacturer's recommendations. These have calculated the dosage for you specifically and should be followed, making sure that you are giving the children dosages for their ages and not adult doses. The only time this can be altered would be if you are under the direct observation from a medical professional that has given specific directions, which you should follow. This is especially important when it comes to children, as excess dosage can harm them (like any medication) if not followed directly. The plus side to this is when you are using a good whole food supplement, it is less likely to happen, because it is like consuming a large amount of food. This definitely isn't a reason to overconsume, as many have the thought process that if a little helps, a lot will really make you better. Please do not fall into this trap, because not all vitamins are water soluble and can build up over time in our body, which could poison or kill someone, especially the little ones if they get too much. Use what is directed on the bottle and, depending on the age, make sure you cut it in half or thirds for the little ones to be safe. Every little bit that they get into their system will help them, so it is better to err on the lower side than take too much and harm them. Again, the warning is not to fear supplements, but to respect what is offered to support your body by taking the dose that has been given as a recommendation.

Since the inside of our body is well covered with good nutrition, plenty of water, and good sources of supplements, we now need to take the time to address the outside and what we can do to help in every aspect of our well-being. This brings us to a very strong topic of essential oils. Some people have found that they love them, while some do not appreciate them. Looking into their benefits, they can be used to enhance great health outcomes. Think of everything you are putting into your body to help make sure it is functioning properly. If that works from the inside out, consider if you could help from the outside of your body to the inside. It seems that you could be even more effective.

Remember, it was mentioned how some may have the mentality that a few supplements work well, so why not take a lot of them? Why not take another approach and think supplements work good from the inside out, and essential oils can work from the outside in? That is the best explanation that can be given for essential oils and how they might help you and your family. Another approach I like to think of for essential oils is the point that some children cannot stand swallowing pills, and you fight them every single day to get them down. What if you could rub essential oils on the bottom of their feet or neck and get similar results? This would help reduce the risk of having them fight you all the time, but yet you are helping them as much as you can.

Not all essential oils are created equal. This should not come to you as a surprise. As was mentioned in the supplement section, they are not regulated by the FDA. This unfortunately leaves the door open for a lot of different varieties and much misunderstanding on what you should do and how you should do it. The first thing you want to do is see if it states 100% therapeutic-grade oils. Just by stating that it is 100% pure can be misleading, since they can be marketed as 100% pure when they have a few drops of pure oil and then the rest of the bottle is filled with cheap synthetic fillers. If it does not state that it is 100% therapeutic grade oil, then you should stay completely away from them. Also, smell them before you buy and see if you can distinctly smell the real product. If you smell several brands, this will become clearer to you.

The major role of essential oils is to place them on your body and let them work through the skin into the bloodstream, rendering them very effective. But like supplements, some essential oil companies are there to sell to the multitudes. So they cheaply fill their bottles with synthetic fillers and then place a couple of drops of essential oils in them. They then call them pure oil and sell it at a fraction of the cost. One question I would ask you is, would you rub fake oil on the bottom of your child's feet or neck? You need to obtain true oils that are extracted straight from the plant to be truly pure. When you use them, you can tell there is a huge difference. We don't know where these filler oils come from and we are trying to eliminate toxins, not introduce more into the body. Another way to test is to put a drop of oil on a piece of paper and see which oil leaves an oil spot in the end. The true oil will not leave a residue and will come out clear. Also, look at the price again. How can one bottle of essential oils be $30-$40, and the same oil along with four others in the same box be $5? This makes things really simple in trying to understand what is real and what is fake. If you aren't comfortable with trying to figure all that out and knowing what is real and fake, contact a couple of the representatives of the main companies and see where their oil is extracted from. These oils come from all over and are extracted and distilled from the plants, which makes them much more suitable for human exposure. However, it will make them that much more expensive because of the process. Fillers are cheap and make cheap products. So, once again you must know the products by reading the labels and understanding them.

Once we have figured out how to make sure that we are purchasing pure essential oils and what to watch out for—what is next? Deciding what to use and when to use it can be confusing and hard to follow. There are lots of different oils out there, and it can become very overwhelming without truly understanding what to buy and why to buy it. First, most oils should be applied to the outside and not ingested. However, there are a few brands out there that do have pure product and allow you to be able to swallow the oils or put them in water. Make sure you consult the companies you are purchasing these oils from to make sure they are ones that you can ingest, and never allow a child to ingest oils unless instructed to by a professional that has experience with that particular brand. When applying the oils to a child or someone that has sensitive skin, it is always advised that you place a carrier oil with the essential oils to dilute it down. This can be done by placing a few drops of oil in your palm of your hand and dropping a few more drops of fractionated coconut oil with it, stirring it around in your palm before applying it. The other options would be to get roller bottles that are glass bottles with a roller on the top. Then you can mix 10–20 drops of the essential oil and then fill the rest of the bottle with the carrier oil, such as fractionated coconut oil, and shake it up. This then makes it easy to apply when you need it multiple times throughout the day. Convenience is key when raising a family, and we need to do all that we can to make sure it is accessible and ready to go when we need it.

Application for essential oils can be very easy to treat and make it easier for reapplication throughout the day. It depends on what is going on, but it has been found most effective to keep applying oils every 2-3 hours every day during acute situations such as the cold, flu, congestion, diarrhea, constipation, or tight muscles. The two main locations for applying the immune boosting oils are the bottom of the feet and the back of the neck. Once you apply the oils to the desired area, rub it in completely like you would lotion or anything else of that nature. Other areas that you could apply oils to for specific issues that could be very beneficial would be the stomach region for constipation, diarrhea, or discomfort; the forehead for headaches or sinus pressure; the neck and throat area for sore throat or cough; and the chest for cough and congestion. There really isn't a specific region that has to be covered, but as close as you can get to the area that is being affected, the better you will be. The oils are absorbed into the body, and then they can pass through the blood/brain barriers so they can directly get into the bloodstream, becoming very effective. From past experience, using oils for diarrhea can help comfort the stomach and make it slow down and stop within a couple of hours. There are some oil companies that have an oil that is a blend that can be applied to bruises and bumps right away, and by the next day they are minimal or nonexistent. This same oil can be applied to the forehead for headaches or sore muscles for a tired parent who has been working all day. That is the nice thing about this—that one oil can be used for multiple things and get results for each one.

Lemon and peppermint make for a good blend when added to honey if one has a sore throat, and you swallow it (make sure it's an oil company that you can do this with). There are also hormone blends that can be very soothing for mother and daughter. Some family favorites are those that help boost the immune system, helping to fight off any sickness such as the flu. These oils are most effective when they are applied morning and night consistently. If someone does come down with a cold or congestion, a respiratory blend can be very helpful to keep it loose. Finally, a calming blend for nighttime is a must have, as it helps the little children sleep better at night. It is very simple to use; apply the oils on their back, bottom of the feet, and the neck region before they go to bed each night. This makes a huge difference, especially in our young ones and how they sleep at night. These same ones can be used for anxiety and stress to relax one before a test or during excess homework.

If you don't feel comfortable applying oils to yourself or chil-dren, consider getting a diffuser and letting it go into the air at night while they sleep. When we have sickness exposure or present, we run our diffusers all the time to combat this, and I have to say that I cannot remember the last time we have had major sickness. We aren't exempt from becoming sick, but we are easily able to fight it with oils and supplements, and it helps keep the symptoms mild so everyone can be back to normal soon.

There are a lot of oils that weren't covered, and it will come down to what brand you get and what you are advised to use. Don't be afraid to reach for any of the oils that are mentioned; just keep in mind that frugality is not something you want to do with essential oils. You want to get a good resource and stick with it when using them. Also, test out a small area on the bottom of the feet to make sure that none of your children will have a sensitive reaction to the oils. It does happen from time to time, and such reactions need to be noted so we don't irritate the skin. If at any time you see a rash or something changing in their skin or on your own, stop using the oils for a period of time and make sure it goes away. Not all skin can handle the pure exposure of the oils, but overall, most can and should be used regularly. If you have someone that has sensitive skin, make sure you are using a carrier oil, such as fractionated coconut oil, to reduce the strength for these individuals. This is also important for children, as their skin cannot handle the direct contact and may cause a harsh burning sensation when applied. Overall, the oils are very safe and can be used over and over in hopes that we can reduce or eliminate our trips to the doctor, and have good and healthy children and families.

The last two topics of herbs and tinctures will be considered together, as they go hand in hand given that most tinctures are made with herbs. This section will be limited, as it is best that you seek the advice of a true herbalist that has experience with herbs and can help give advice on proper dosage.

Tinctures are created from herbs with either an alcohol or glycerol base and are used for the valued nutrients from the herbs. It is advised that you use caution with these, as many of them are alcohol-based and really not the best for children. So, if you are going to venture into this area, consider getting the glycerol-based tinctures. Make sure that you follow the proper dosage guidelines that are given. Because of the breakdown that may happen, it will be harder to distinguish the actual dose that a child should have. The benefit of a tincture is that it can get directly absorbed into the bloodstream through the mouth and be very effective faster. It may be advised not to consume a large variety, but stick with the plan that an herbalist has designed based on your symptoms or how they assessed you or your children. This way, you will make certain that they know what is going on, and if ill symptoms occur, they can be followed up with.

Of the alternative medicine options, it is best to conclude that they can be extremely helpful and, more importantly, can be taken as a preventative. Imagine if you could reduce the sickness of your children or yourself throughout the year by taking something that you have on hand and applying it or swallowing it. There are so many different options, and when you buy a good quality source, you can rest assured that your body can utilize it and absorb it properly. It should be reminded that we need to make sure the rest of our body is in check and that we have our digestive system working properly so we can absorb these high-quality nutrients. If you are ever required to take a medication, it would be best to always follow that up with a good probiotic or increased level to make sure any damaging effects can be repaired. If not, that is where damage can lead to increased inflammation, which then leads to continued leakage in the gut, not allowing us to pull and absorb the good nutrients from the supplements.

Take time to read the labels, and once you find a good source of alternative medicine, stay with it and continue to let it work as it should. Jumping from one company to another can slow down the progress, and not allowing the time your body needs to heal and repair will leave you feeling frustrated, believing that the nutrients are ineffective. Always know that any form of natural medicine takes time to get into the body and to build up in an effective way. These aren't like the traditional drugs, where you take a week and you feel a night-and-day difference. They take a long time, and to be fair, have a better response as a result because it takes a slower process to build up. Give it the time it needs to determine if something works or not. Don't just toss it out, but give weeks to a month (or longer) to really let it run its course. Then you can evaluate and make that determination if further action is needed. Consider your options, buy good quality, follow the directions, and you should see the results in yourself and children.

"If you think compliance is expensive—try non-compliance."

- Paul McNulty

12

COMPLIANCE

Follow the rules or not?

THIS SECTION WASN'T going to be included in this book, as it was going to be discussed at a later point with a follow-up book. However, the topic continues to come up and be a problem that should be discussed and talked through a little. Look out for another book that will go into a deeper discussion on this topic and why it is so important to follow through with what is recommended and actually do what you learn as you go along. There is no value in reading or listening to any discussion if you don't wish to follow some of the guidelines that are expressed here.

It has been mentioned over and over that you need to take baby steps to achieve living a healthy lifestyle. That is exactly what needs to be done, and you must be committed to making it happen not just for today, but for a lifetime. Lifestyle changes don't mean trying it for a day or week, finding that it is too hard to do, and then going back to unhealthy ways of life. If you seek the advice from someone who is knowledgeable in health and wellness, then follow through with what they are recommending.

You cannot get well by doing it for a day or two, or even up to a week or two, and expect a miracle of changes in the way you feel. As a society, we have depended on the model that you just take a pill and you will be healed and feel great again. We have to get away from this thought process and understand that good health takes time to accomplish and hard work to keep up.

"IT IS BETTER TO MAKE MANY SMALL STEPS IN THE RIGHT DIRECTION THAN TO MAKE A GREAT LEAP FORWARD ONLY TO STUMBLE BACKWARD."
PROVERB

We need to break away from the model that medicine will cure it all. We have to take responsibility for our health and the health of our family. We can't depend on the medical system to provide one pill that fixes all. We need to avoid the model that if you don't feel better after one day with a good diet and supplements, it's not working. Remember one thing, how long did it take you to get to this point of not feeling well? It will take that same amount of time, if not longer, to regain what you have lost in wellness. Are you willing to put in that time for a lifetime, or would you rather have that easy fix so you don't have to do anything? So many get discouraged a few days in and give up with no results, then turn right back to their old ways of unhealthy living. The medical realm is destroying us, and we are all becoming reliant on that quick model which damages us in the end.

If you don't understand what is being presented here, consider how many different weight loss programs you have seen people go through where they either lose the weight over time, or they give up half way through and just accept the way they are, not wanting to go through the pain of losing it all.

The other option is that they work so hard trying to get it all off and reach their goal, then gain it all back because so many of us are not willing to work hard, learn the value of eating well, and then implement this lifestyle for our entire life. We want to do this for a short time and then get back to "normal." Normal is living a life that we enjoy and feel a stability every day that we do it. Eating well and staying healthy can be normal if we learn how to do this and maintain it.

Being healthy part time doesn't work at all. Taking baby steps to gain the lifetime of eating and being healthy is a plan that can be followed and should be considered. Part-time healthy is exactly what it sounds like and you get part-time results. Consider someone working for you that is only part time. They may enjoy what they do and work hard, but do they truly have the interest of the company in mind while they are doing it? Not so much, because they only put in part of their time, where someone that is present every day and puts the time in has a bigger investment and is more determined to succeed and make sure the company succeeds. There is always the exception to the rule but, in the end, it is a great guide we can follow. It will never work if you plan on getting healthy for a short amount of time and then go back to your old habits. It will not work if you eat healthy most of the time, but indulge in desserts and sugars off and on when you "have to have them." We all like to be rewarded for eating well and being healthy, but that shouldn't be an indulgence to reward yourself. Most of the time when someone does this, they continue to do it over and over again, giving themselves an excuse every time to "cheat" a little because they deserve it. Their family has done so well that they can have one time to celebrate and eat fast food. This only creates a craving in your mouth and body for more, and you already have justified it, giving yourself the go-ahead to do it again. Holding strong to your true desires will instill a more powerful outcome long-term, and gives your kids understanding that excuses will get you nowhere in life. So why not use it for that purpose and hold strong to eating well and being well? This can go for eating or exercising—always trying to do what you can to be healthy.

Another example is that there are some diet programs that allow you a "cheat" day or time. When has this ever been a good thing, and why do so many people thrive after that one day? One would very seldom hear someone say that they used up their vegetable day, but certainly they have hit every one of their cheat days. The sad part about this is that soon cheat days happen more and more, and they keep promising to themselves that they will make it up later in the week, but later never comes. One last thought on that is, what kind of message do we send to our kids when we say that we are on a cheat day and that's okay? But when they want to cheat on schoolwork or a game, that is definitely out of the question. How this works one time, but not another time, is what does not make sense. This is no indication that it is easy to make these changes, but go back to why you are truly doing it and what you truly want for your family.

The last thing that needs to be expressed is the point that if you want to seek advice because something isn't right, then follow through with it. So often, we seek the advice from some-one we read or talk with and then we go home and decide we didn't like what we heard, so we go seek advice from someone else. Let's face the fact that everyone has their own way of doing something, and in the end it may all work, but if we don't put the time in to see it through, it won't work out. We have wasted all of our time and the time of others if we seek their advice. But in the end, we decide to do nothing. Consider that if you went to them in the beginning, you obviously had enough respect to value what they had to tell you. Trying what they said for a day or two (or even a week) doesn't always work, and you move on to the next person. This does not give their method a true and honest effort, and of course will not be successful if you did not give it the time that it needed to be successful.

"IT'S NEVER TOO EARLY OR TOO LATE TO WORK TOWARDS BEING THE HEALTHIEST YOU."

GET HEALTHY

As was mentioned at the start of this, health takes time, even in a trauma situation, so we have to allow that time to heal. Going from person to person and not allowing anything to work does not heal the body. In fact, it hinders the healing process and can do more damage in the end. The opposite can be said that if we are following someone's advice and things are not getting better over a longer period of time, and we have done everything they stated exactly. Then, by all means, it is time to seek other advice and avenues to resolve the issue. This is not what is being discussed, and it is fully advised that if you don't get desired results and you have spent months honestly working with their directives, then you need to move on to someone or something else. Not every model will work for every person, just as not every pill will fit every symptom, and we have to recognize that as well. Just use this as a general rule and ask yourself: "Have I followed all of the directions that they gave me? Have I taken exactly what they told me to take, and at what times they told me? Have I removed everything from my diet they told me to do?" If you have dotted all your "i's" and crossed all your "t's" for several months and see absolutely no results or things have gotten progressively worse, then progress to the next person. Until then, stay focused and determined on doing what you have set out to do.

"NUTRITION ISN'T JUST ABOUT EATING, IT'S ABOUT LEARNING TO LIVE."
PATRICIA COMPTTON

It seems that so few of us are willing to follow through when it comes to our health. Supplements or dietary changes take time, and will need to be processed over time at the dosage that is recommended. If we decide to take matters into our own hands and cut the dose or enhance the dose, we are taking a risk that none of us should. Those that have given us the recommendations know our history and can understand what contradictions come along with too much or too little. If we don't know what we should be taking because we found it at a store, then follow the directions on the bottle until guided otherwise. Don't follow the guidance of someone that is taking it, but follow what is tested and advised. Don't ever use the idea that "A little is good, so if I take a lot then it should be even better." This can harm you, as some vitamins are fat soluble and you can overdose on them, especially young children. The same with taking only half a dose. The recommended dose has been set up to be effective, so follow through with it and do what is advised so that you get the results. So many want to cut the dose and make it last because it is so expensive, but then complain that they don't get the results they are looking for. The dose has been set up to give you what you need when you need it. If you complain that you aren't getting the results you want and you have a full bottle at the end of the month when you should be ordering more, then there is your problem. It isn't the supplement, it is not the program, it is your lack of responsibility to fulfill what was asked of you to get well. Don't put any blame on anyone who is helping you when you did not help yourself.

Compliance is key to changing your lifestyle, and if you do exactly what you are advised or what you read, you will see results. It does not have to be specifically one program or information or another; just following through will give you some kind of results. Understand that getting progressively worse did not happen right away, so make note of the little changes that happen. This means the very little changes that happen. If your child has a behavioral outbreak, make note of when it happens, and keep track of that. Before you started, were they happening several times a week, and now they are down to a half of that? Think about diet changes; if you are wanting to lose weight, it takes a pound or two at a time. You did not wake up one day fifty pounds overweight, and the same applies for losing that weight. Note how much you lose each week, not daily, and consistently weigh every week at the same time if possible. This will show your progress the most, and you can accurately depict what is going on. If your child is struggling in school, then note the small changes, even in grades, as you go along. There are always markers in which we can make little progress, and any time you grow a little you are making advances to better health. Always remember, it takes time to achieve greatness, and the time well spent will be time you have earned longer with your family and for them to feel and do well.

"The doctor of the future will no longer
treat the human frame with drugs, but rather
will cure and prevent disease with nutrition."

- Thomas Edison

FAREWELL!

This is not a goodbye, but a hope
you will carry on the future.

THIS BOOK IS COMING to a close, and as most of us would probably like to express, we never want to end or say that final goodbye. But with all good things we have to realize that we have work to do and many thoughts that need to be processed. We hope that as you go through this book, you have discovered good information, but most importantly, valuable tips that you can take with you as you move forward. It was referenced several times throughout the book that many good things take time and patience to achieve, and a truly good healthy lifestyle is one of them. The reason we have found ourselves even having this conversation is that we have become dependent on the conveniences of life, and we need to take a step back and realize that even though these have made our life simpler, they come with a price for our health.

There are many thought processes out there, and you may find that some of the things that are talked about in this book are too complex for your family. The important thing you need to realize is that we won't put something into motion if we feel it is too complex. So, just like any other resource out there, take as much information as you can and adapt as much as you can, but realize not every application will apply to every situation. It doesn't matter what book you read or how many people it has helped; at the end of the day, if it isn't a simple and practical application for your family, then it may not work. Take what works and do what you can to make the most changes you can to be successful. Every little nugget you can pull away may be a little step closer, and you will instill in your children the value of eating well and, in the end, feeling well.

We are too busy in our life to make that perfect change and hand that perfect lifestyle down to our children, and let's be real, life isn't perfect. We can come up with thousands of excuses, and that tends to happen on a regular basis if we are in tune with what we want for our family. We can let the business of life get the best of us and find a reason why easy and fast foods are so much more convenient. A thought that has been expressed over time and especially now is that "I can't change the way my kids eat," and how true it is today. But you can make a difference, and just like any of the core values you try to teach our kids, they will go back to it someday.

These things don't leave their internal mind, and even I myself look back and can see the things that we did as kids still shine through as lessons we learned. We naturally pass them on to our children, and they remember them and pass them on to their children. Sure, we all know there are things that we maybe don't see as necessary and some traditions that seemed a little funny that we no longer take part in, but overall, the core concepts and values do get passed on from generation to generation. The same can be said with our health and well-being, and how we look at eating and taking care of our bodies through proper nutrition and exercise can be communicated to our children so they can reflect back on it. There will be times that they may wander off and consume daily fast food and let go of their body, but if you have taken the time to really help them understand the value of good eating and wellness habits at a young age, they will return to them. We even find ourselves reflecting on how we've slipped and need to clean things up a bit, but we know what we have to do. If they are never taught what we know and what our grandparents knew, or even what we have learned, they won't have anything to go back to. Why not take this time now and shape and mold them with the knowledge of good nutrition and valuable habits of keeping our body in good shape? What they do as kids and into early adulthood will have a lasting impact on their older years.

The last comment that needs to be expressed is the point that we all die someday. Because of this, many have shared that they want to eat and do whatever they want to enjoy their life now. We will all die someday is a true statement. There is no changing that, but consider one thing—would you want to die suffering from a condition for months or years, with someone caring for you all the time and you losing all dignity? Or would you like to make the decision to take care of yourself now to ensure that you can live the happiest active life in the future? Really think about that. Even worse, would you like to outlive your children and bury each of them because you didn't take the time to help them understand the importance of taking care of themselves?

We all know that some diseases cannot be controlled and decreases our life expectancy, but proper nutrition can play a bigger role in caring for ourselves and reducing the likelihood of premature death, even with the worst diseases. We all know this, but we seem to lose this focus and spend our time enjoying what we want, when we want, and don't realize we may suffer more in the future. None of us want that, and we especially don't want that for our children. Give your children something they can inherit and pass on for many years to come; something you can be proud of, knowing you made a difference in the world. If we could simply make a little change in our lives, we can make a little change in our children's lives, which then can make a difference in their children's lives. In doing so, we can change the world a little at a time. It doesn't have to be hard, but it can be simple steps at first that can make the biggest difference and impact in the future.

As you sit here and really ponder what you can do as an individual, take just an extra second and really create a simple way that you can make a little change. This book isn't all-inclusive and there is a lot more that could be explained and discussed. This book isn't here to treat anyone or cure diseases. It is just a simple guide to take a family small or large and help them to implement lifestyle changes to make a healthier difference in their life. You don't have to agree with everything that is written here or support all the changes; just taking a little bit here and there that is valuable to you and your family can make all the difference in the end. The world is filled with excuses. If we keep living every single day with these excuses, we won't make the changes we want. Our children are dying at such a young age or suffering diseases they should not be suffering from because we want to live in a world of convenience and excuses. We want to live the way we want to live, when in return we are killing ourselves and our children. It isn't easy to make these changes, but within 3-4 weeks habits can be formed and we can implement these changes. Can we all start by making a simple change one habit at a time, and implement them for our children for years to come? It comes down to using the knowledge we learn to do better and passing it on, which may make all the difference in the future.

RESOURCES

*These are additional resources that can be helpful and ones that I utilized in this book.

Kharrazian, D. (2013). Why Isn't My Brain Working? Amsterdam University Press.

Osborne, P. (2016). No Grain, No Pain. Adfo Books.

Melillo, R. (2009). Disconnected Kids. Perigee Book.

Wilson, J. L., & Smart Publications. (2001). Adrenal Fatigue. Smart Publications.

Zielinski, D. E. C., & DC, E. Z. (2018). The Healing Power of Essential Oils. Potter/Ten Speed/Harmony/Rodale.

Hyman, M. (2017). Broken Brain Series. Hyman Digital

Nab, G. (2016) 1 degree of Change, Standard Process

Shojai, P. (2019) Interconnected Series, Interconnected Media LLC

globalhealingcenter.com

sunwarrior.com/healthhub

cdc.gov/obesity/childhood/index.html

who.int/maternal_child_adolescent/topics/child/imci/en/

To purchase *Easy Cooking Healthy Eating,* please fill out this form and mail it along with your cash or check to:

Nu-Atrics
211 W. Willow St.
Fairbury, IL 61739
(309) 807-3323

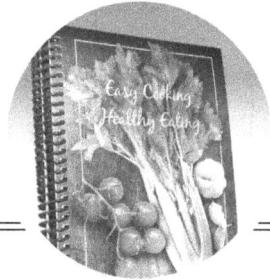

Make checks payable to: Nu-Atrics.

CUSTOMER INFO

NAME

ADDRESS

CITY   ST   ZIP

PHONE

☐ CASH

SHIP TO ADDRESS

☐ CHECK

NAME

ADDRESS

CITY   ST   ZIP

ITEM	QTY	PRICE (INCLUDING SHIPPING)	TOTAL
COOKBOOK		$15/EA	

CALL FOR LARGE ORDER DISCOUNTS

ACKNOWLEDGMENTS

To my amazing wife Shawna and my five beautiful children, Micah, Audrey, Kaden, Brynlee, and Treyson, who never lost hope that I would complete this book. They realize the importance of what this book expresses and wanted to see it in the hands of so many around the world. If it wasn't for their sacrifice and continued support, this would never have been a reality.

To Jonathan and Nancy Laudon and their team that recognized the vision that we had in spreading the word of good nutrition for the entire family, thank you for the unlimited support you provided during this process and the ability to work so closely together.

To Chelsea Rosario, for the outstanding design work and the many ideas you shared during this process. It was a pleasure working with you on it and I hope for many more in the future.

www.ingramcontent.com/pod-product-compliance
Lightning Source LLC
Chambersburg PA
CBHW062058270326
41931CB00013B/3130